CONTENTS

Foreword to this Edition

Since this book was written, HRT has become more widely prescribed and about one in four women now start taking HRT when they reach the menopause. However, many give up after quite a short time. One of the main reasons for this is that they do not like having to put up with monthly bleeds – 'periods' – again. So far, Livial has been the only HRT offering 'bleed-free' cycles but now two new therapies which do so – Kliofem and Premique – are available and others are in the pipeline. This form of HRT is known as 'continuous combined therapy'. It is taken as one daily tablet containing a small amount of oestrogen as well as a low dose of progestogen which prevents a build up of the womb lining. Although bleeding and spotting are common to begin with, many women find that, after a few months' use, the light spotting there may still be is acceptable and certainly preferable to a heavier monthly bleed – 'period'. Possible pre-menstrual-type side effects, such as breast tenderness, also tend to improve. Like Livial, this type of HRT should not be started until at least one year after the woman's last natural period.

One advantage of a new oestrogen-containing patch called Evorel and others of the matrix type, is that they are less likely to cause skin-sensitive reactions. They are also less noticeable than some other patches and tend to stay on better. Another new oestrogen patch, Progynova TS, only needs changing once a week instead of twice and is said to be almost invisible.

Oestrogel is another new HRT. With this, a measured amount of oestrogen-containing cream is rubbed into the skin each day – anywhere except onto the breast or around the vagina. It is then absorbed into the blood stream. Skin reactions to the cream are said to be rare. With both the new patches and the cream, progestogen tablets will need to be taken for the last 12 days of the cycle to produce a bleed if the woman has not had a hysterectomy. Yet another option now on offer is Tridestra – a regime of oestrogen and progestogen tablets producing a 'period' only once in three months.

So, with these new developments and others which will surely follow, it is becoming ever easier for women to enjoy the benefits of HRT without the drawbacks.

Dr. Mike Smith's Postbag
HRT

DR MIKE SMITH is an NHS Director of Public Health Medicine and President of the Association of Broadcasting Doctors. He was the Chief Medical Officer of the Family Planning Association 1970–75 and their Honorary Medical Adviser 1975–90. He is an elected member of the FPA's National Executive Committee and a member of the advisory panel of both the National Food Safety Advisory Centre and the British Association of Continence Care. For many years he has been a 'resident' expert guest on BBC2's Jimmy Young Programme, LBC's Nightline and the medical columnist/editor for *Woman's Own*. Between 1980 and 1984 he presented BBC1's health series 'Looking Good, Feeling Fit' and from 1988–90 he was the expert guest on SKY TV's 'Sky by Day'. In April 1991, he was voted the TV and Radio Doctors' 'Expert's Expert' in the *Observer* magazine's series.

His other books include *Birth Control*, *How to Save Your Child's Life*, *A New Dictionary of Symptoms* and *Dr Mike Smith's Handbook of Over-The-Counter Medicines*.

IONA SMITH is a qualified nurse, specialising in Family Planning and the menopause. She is also a successful journalist. For many years she wrote the medical page and answered reader's letters for *Woman's Weekly* magazine. She therefore has special knowledge and understanding of the problems that concern women. She is married to Dr Mike Smith and they have three grown-up children.

Also in *Dr Mike Smith's Postbag* series:

IONA SMITH

DR MIKE
SMITH'S
POSTBAG

HRT

WITH MARGARET ROOKE

KYLE CATHIE LIMITED

This edition published 1996

First published 1993 by
Kyle Cathie Limited
20 Vauxhall Bridge Road
London SW1V 2SA

ISBN 1 85626 229 4

A CIP catalogue record for this title
is available from the British Library

Typeset by DP Photosetting, Aylesbury, Bucks
Printed and bound in Great Britain by Cox & Wyman Ltd., Reading, Berkshire

INTRODUCTION

In times gone by menopausal misery was not a great problem for women – they tended not to live that long! Even at the beginning of this century the average age a woman could hope to reach was somewhere between forty and fifty. So the change she faced was not from menstruation and fertility to the menopause but something rather more drastic . . .

The average age of the menopause has hardly altered in the past century – it's still somewhere between forty-nine and fifty-one – but a hundred years ago less than one in three women reached the menopause while today the figure is around nine out of ten.

These days women are likely to live until they're eighty, longer than men in fact. Older women make up around a fifth of our population and are playing a more and more important part in the public world. From politicians to industrialists, to actresses and artists, they're becoming more visual and more prominent. They have more choice in their private lives too. At around the time their periods are stopping some are becoming grandmothers while others are becoming mothers for the first time.

It's strange to think their forebears were those being referred to in this both hilarious and sad extract from a book published in the 1920s called *Everybody's Family Doctor*, quoted in a newspaper article we came across the other day. Obviously a reference book of stature of its time, it says under 'Menopause':

Some women, especially those of neurotic temperament, become unable to control their emotions. These women may be such a nuisance that they have to be shut up in institutions where they can be cared for by specially trained nurses ... Their behaviour, too, may cause the break-up of a home that has hitherto been happy. Forbearance on the part of the husband may tide over this period until the wife returns to a more normal frame of mind.

Thankfully these days we have a rather less extreme and very much more sympathetic view of the effects the menopause may have. We take seriously the symptoms that were, until recently, dismissed as 'unimportant' and 'just something that has to be lived with' – from insomnia, nausea and headaches to hot flushes, vaginal dryness, mood swings, depression and anxiety. True, they may not require radical surgery and they may not be life-threatening (although depression can lead one to feel very, very low indeed) but they can still cause huge amounts of discomfort, pain, worry, embarrassment, low self-esteem and sadness.

Nowadays we're willing and able to talk about a part of women's lives that was taboo, that was never acknowledged or spoken about, and in doing this the positive side of the menopause is becoming apparent. As the channels of communication have opened, more and more women are telling us in their letters how they've moved from feeling negatively about leaving their youth and fertility behind them to looking positively at what the rest of their life may have to offer. And they're determined to have the energy and good health to live it to the full. Often we feel more zest and drive coming from their words than we do from those of many younger correspondents.

The menopause is a complex and confusing period for most women and often occurs at the same time as other big changes. It may be the time when children leave home or when conflicts with them are greatly increased. It may be a time of illness for themselves or their family or friends, or of caring for dependent parents on a full- or part-time basis. It may be a time of bereavement, of losing parents and other elderly relatives. It may be a time of early retirement or redundancy and the changes in finances and status and lifestyle these bring.

While all this is happening their bodies decide to give them even more to think about and cope with. The ovaries stop functioning and the level of the hormone oestrogen which they produce falls by four or five times. This means that tissues dependent on oestrogen become deficient in the hormone and suffer because of it. The skin becomes drier and hair thinner. The vaginal walls, too, become thinner and less lubricated and the vulva may be sore. Also breasts become less full and firm. Amongst other symptoms, women may also suffer pains in the joints and night sweats and, as we've already mentioned, the dreaded hot flushes.

Not every woman will experience all of this. As a rough guide, up to a third will experience a very bad menopause, a third will find their symptoms unpleasant but not severe and others will hardly notice the change.

However the lack of oestrogen has longer-term physical effects. Bones need the hormone for without it osteoporosis can take hold, as the bones become fragile and porous and may be fractured by even a slight fall. Oestrogen is also beneficial for the heart and cardiovascular system. In addition and, some experts feel, more importantly, without the hormone women lose their advantages over men in protection against heart disease and strokes.

The more immediate unpleasant effects of the menopause are sometimes seen as an inevitable part of middle age that has to be coped with alone. We've known many women who stand up for themselves generally in life and are very strong and powerful figures but who suffered their menopause in silence, not asking for help, just soldiering through. Yes, the menopause is a natural part of being a woman – but then periods are natural too and we do our best to make them more bearable with painkillers, Oil of Evening Primrose, warm baths and relaxation techniques.

There are, similarly, many different ways to relieve menopausal problems and we've outlined them in this book. However our main focus is on one way in particular, Hormone Replacement Therapy.

Those whose only knowledge of HRT has been gained through skim-reading popular newspapers may have the impression that this is the medication exclusively supplied to glamorous, lipsticked film and television stars, who reveal how they've regained their youth and glossy hair and who are delighted to find they have the same sexual needs as their latest young lover. But the truth is that HRT is an accepted, respected part of preventative medicine, taken by hundreds of thousands of women around the world to replenish their hormone levels during and after the menopause. As hormone levels are raised, the aim is that women will no longer suffer unpleasant menopausal symptoms, and the longer-term medical effects of oestrogen deficiency will be curbed.

What is surprising is the length of time that replacing hormones has been available to help women suffering the effects of oestrogen deficiency. Far from a new development in women's health care, implants of oestrogen were first used as long ago as 1938 and the first modern combination pills were prescribed in 1974. This is no flash-in-the-pan miracle cure that's just been produced from nowhere.

However doubts, not always based on fact, still exist about the treatment, and according to your letters even some family doctors lack sound information about the latest research findings and are intimidated by some of the scare stories that exist.

Of course there are risks. There *has* been conflicting evidence, especially about the possibility of an increased likelihood of breast cancer for those taking the combined oestrogen and progestogen form of HRT. And of course it's always better not to take drugs than it is to take them. We have to weigh up risks we know about and just maybe some of the ones we don't. But the benefits can be enormous too.

Mike remembers a women writing to him in great detail about her menopausal symptoms – her insomnia, night sweats, aching joints and her fears that osteoporosis was waiting for her round the corner as she'd seen both her mother and her grandmother suffer with it, losing, it had seemed to them, their independence and dignity. 'I felt as if I couldn't go on and I was bringing the whole family down with me,' she wrote.

> The children were staying out later and later and I think that was partly because they'd never know what sort of mood I'd be in when they got home. My husband was accepting more and more overtime at work and I don't think it was just for the money. When I talked to him about it I realised it was partly to get himself some peace away from me. With HRT I feel so much calmer. I feel a new sense of hope and that life has plenty to offer again.

We always feel it's a shame to present just one solution if a choice exists and we hope you'll be interested in reading about some of the less conventional options too. We believe what's also exciting is the extent to which the diet and lifestyle you choose can affect your health and your body and its response to the changes which will inevitably come its way. Maybe these can also provide longer-term hope and benefits for younger members of your family and friends for whom the menopause may seem a million miles away. Of course they have years stretched in front of them but there's still plenty they can do to keep healthy and ensure as easy a time as possible.

One of the ways we hope they and you will do this is by seeing the menopause not as something negative and depressing but as a natural part of life which does have its good side. No more periods means no more contraceptive worries for a start. It means the beginning of a whole new period of your life – maybe with less responsibilities for looking after children and more time to spend on yourself and to decide what will fulfil and excite you.

For many women the menopause can mean misery but we hope in this book to help you solve physical and emotional predicaments and find your path to a comfortable and satisfying future.

Chapter One
THE MENOPAUSE AND HRT

Your menopause is approaching. Are you looking forward to an active and fulfilling life ahead or are you dreading the changes which are about to take place in your body?

Some women have found their late forties and fifties is the time when they've come into their own, maybe even started a new career. They claim the post-menopausal years can be the best thirty years of your life – and, as we shall see, many believe that Hormone Replacement Therapy must take a great deal of the credit for giving them added vitality and a health and energy boost.

But first we want to look at the menopause itself. It's worth going into this in some detail, especially as it is a time in a woman's life so shrouded in mystery and, depressingly, taboo.

SIGNS AND SYMPTOMS

Menopause literally means the end of menstruation but these days the term is used more generally to cover the whole process of bodily change which can begin three or more years before a woman's periods stop and can carry on for several years afterwards. In the medical profession this is known as the 'climacteric'. However just because there's a medical term doesn't mean we're talking about an illness. Far from it. This is just an inevitable and natural part of every woman's life.

It's not really possible to judge when the first signs of

the menopause will begin. It's been suggested that if you start your periods earlier than average you may find they stop later than average and if you begin them later you may find they stop earlier, but there are no hard and fast rules.

A recent survey carried out by the *Daily Express* and ICM Research found a third of its sample noticing the menopause starting between the ages of forty-six and fifty, with the next most common time between forty-one and forty-five. Medically speaking, fifty is average, forty-five is early, anything before forty is premature.

Some women get no warning at all of the menopause descending, their periods simply stop as suddenly as they started all those years before. But this isn't typical. Usually a woman's periods become scant and the length of time between them gets longer and longer until they finally stop completely. On the other hand, they can sometimes become more heavy than they've been before and very irregular. Some can last so long there are very few clear days between one stopping and the next one starting.

During and after the menopause the body produces less oestrogen than during the fertile years. Oestrogen is the collective name for a group of hormones which are vital for the growth of eggs, for the reproductive process and for the development of the breasts. It maintains the cells of the womb and the vagina and stimulates the production of vaginal mucus which should mean sexual intercourse is pain-free. It also helps fight infection. As I mentioned in the Introduction, it helps prevent heart disease and osteoporosis and also affects the skin, hair, blood, bones, nails and body shape.

The bodily changes which result in the menopause are quite simple. When her periods begin, a girl's body produces an egg every month which can be fertilised by a man's sperm. If it isn't fertilised, the egg is expelled from the body along with the specially prepared womb lining and the extra supply of blood provided by the body to nourish and feed the egg in case it is fertilised. That is menstruation.

When a woman reaches middle age, the body begins to cut down on its production of oestrogen which, as we have seen, is the hormone which supports this ovulation process. This means the womb no longer prepares for fertilisation and periods stop. This whole process may take several years as hormone levels may not be consistent.

There's a more precise reason for the symptoms many women face at the time of the menopause. The pituitary gland and its associated tissues put out hormones into the bloodstream from the time of puberty and these hormones stimulate the ovaries which then produce their own ovarian hormones – both oestrogen and progesterone. At the time of the menopause the ovaries are coming to the end of their reproductive work so they don't respond as readily to the pituitary trigger hormones. The pituitary gland counters this by putting out more trigger hormones – called gonadotrophins – and the high level of these creates the symptoms associated with the menopause.

These symptoms differ from woman to woman. Many find they don't suffer at all while roughly two thirds of women feel some of the symptoms of oestrogen deficiency, for example hot flushes, night sweats, pains in their joints, irritability, bladder problems and tiredness. The symptoms can last for more than two years; in the very unlucky some of them can last for the rest of a woman's life. But, we must stress, they are the *very* unlucky. In all but a tiny percentage of cases there is very definitely light at the end of the tunnel.

The physical and emotional changes faced by women can be as wide-ranging as the hot flushes already mentioned – thirty times a day in the worst cases – constipation, headaches, itching all over, vaginal dryness, dryness of the eyes, visual disturbances, incontinence, hair loss from the scalp, hair growth on the face, weaker muscles and a thinner skin which is more prone to ageing. Energy levels, concentration levels and memory levels drop. Many women find they can't bring themselves to make a simple decision and some forget very basic and routine things. A good night's sleep is a distant memory. Life can be very difficult at home and in relationships and also at work where standards kept to during a career or working lifetime can now seem impossible to maintain. The lack of comprehension and sympathy from others which might result will only add to a sufferer's problems, worse still could be directed inwardly as she impatiently tells herself off for not being able to cope.

Interestingly, there's some debate about whether the psychological signs of the 'menopause' – from tiredness to loss of concentration and irritability – are down to a lack of oestrogen. This is because women in the developing world don't appear to suffer these same symptoms – and the custom in these countries is for women to celebrate their menopause rather than to dread it. Often the menopause gives these women an increase in standing and stature and sometimes an added freedom to mix with men more widely than before. So who knows to what degree the way our society values youth so highly and treats old age so poorly causes our more depressive menopausal symptoms?

There are many bodily changes. At the time of the menopause the breasts lose some of the fat just underneath the skin and the mammary gland tissue, which produces breast milk, shrinks. Fat moves to the waist and hips. As well as vaginal dryness, which is caused by a diminishing of vaginal secretions, the tissues of the vagina and vulva lose their elasticity and become thinner, adding to the problem of painful intercourse. Unfortunately this may also lead to urinary problems such as cystitis and frequency because the thinness of the vagina and vulva means there's less of a cushioning effect during intercourse and so the tube through which the urine passes – the urethra – can get bruised.

A questionnaire filled in by *Woman's Weekly* readers gave some indication of the extent to which all aspects of a woman's life may be affected by the menopause. (Remember this survey will have been completed by women with a specific interest in menopausal symptoms and so are more likely to have suffered rather than had an easy path.) Of four thousand replies received by the magazine, 88 per cent complained of hot flushes, by a long way the most common symptom. For women in their early to mid-fifties the figure rose to 93 per cent of respondents. Night sweats were the second most common symptom reported – 78 per cent said they suffered from them, with some women waking ten times a night.

Nearly 70 per cent said they were irritable and moody, 44 per cent said they suffered from dizziness and 41 per cent from palpitations. A third said they had sexual problems resulting from their menopausal symptoms. Sexual problems together with irritability had the biggest adverse effects on their relationships. Other problems included headaches, lack of confidence, exhaustion and aching joints.

There must be some advantages with these bodily changes, we hear you cry. Well, as we've already mentioned, there's the end to periods, though with most types of HRT bleeding will return. There's a possible decreased risk of breast cancer as the body produces less oestrogen, but then with long-term HRT the risk may slightly increase again. Sometimes you just can't win. At least the need for contraception has gone and that can be a big benefit for a couple's sex life, especially if one or other of you has never been totally happy with the form of contraception you use.

We find it quite astonishing, bearing in mind that every woman who survives to middle age goes through a menopause and bearing in mind how widespread the pain and discomfort of these symptoms can be, just how little the condition is talked about even in the 1990s. Before the advent of HRT and all the publicity surrounding it, the word 'menopause' was barely spoken in public and rarely mentioned even between women.

We feel this is one of the reasons why there are still so many gaps in knowledge about this important time in women's lives, even among women who take an interest in their health.

Did you know, for example, that every female starts life with an incredible seven million eggs inside her and she'll never manufacture any more? When she's born that amount has reduced to two million and from here the numbers go downhill all the way. By the time her periods start she will probably have just 300,000 eggs left and that number will become smaller and smaller as the years go by. Of course the occasional egg will be fertilised and grow into a baby, many will be lost during the ovulation process when they're not fertilised, and many more will be lost through natural degeneration. So by the age of fifty a woman is likely to have run out of eggs. However she can lose them even more rapidly. Her egg supply can have dried up by the age of forty or thirty, and in rare cases twenty or earlier still.

PREMATURE MENOPAUSE

There are many different theories about why some women lose eggs more rapidly than others but no one has come forward with a definite cause for the premature menopause which is entirely spontaneous, that is it hasn't been influenced by outside interference. What we can be sure about is that nothing the woman herself has done will be responsible, although we know from letters we receive that many women do blame themselves and falsely target abortions or miscarriages as the reason for their fertility coming to a close.

There are some known circumstances which can trigger a very early menopause. If her ovaries are 'inflamed' this can lead the woman to develop antibodies which will go on to destroy the ovaries. Also, if the ovaries have to be removed because the woman is suffering from a disease – a procedure known as an oopherectomy – this causes the menopause. Another cause is chemotherapy and radiotherapy – the ovaries can be irreversibly damaged by these treatments and, again, this will result in a premature menopause.

If the menopause is early this means not only that a woman has fewer years in which to have a baby, but also fewer years of benefit from natural oestrogen supplies and so is more likely to suffer from early and serious osteoporosis and also secondary osteoarthritis. Pregnancy isn't totally out of the question after a premature menopause but the only method of conception that can be tried is a test-tube technique using an egg from a donor as the woman has no eggs of her own left. Occasionally women find themselves pregnant without using this method, to their total surprise. What might have happened here is that they were suffering from what's known as Resistant Ovaries Syndrome. This means they think they have had the menopause – their periods stop and they have other symptoms normally associated with the change – but what's actually happened is that their ovaries aren't responding to natural hormonal stimulation. If they start taking HRT, the additional hormones in the therapy lead to fertility being stimulated in a way that's little understood. It's important not to raise your hopes if you desperately want a baby and are now wondering whether you might still have a chance. Resistant Ovaries Syndrome is rare and is readily diagnosed by a specialist so a second opinion would be thought wise by most doctors.

Olivia

Olivia, a mother of two, suffered from a very premature menopause when she was thirty-two. She'd had an ovary removed ten years before and then three years ago, surgeons operating on her remaining ovary to remove a cyst decided they had to take that ovary out as well.

> I didn't realise what that meant and what a dramatic effect this would have on me when I came round and they told me what they'd done. I didn't realise that by taking out my ovaries they'd started my menopause. It never crossed my mind in my early thirties. I went through hot flushes not knowing what was happening, not knowing why I couldn't sleep. Then someone made a passing remark about the menopause and suddenly I realised.
>
> I rang my surgeon up and I had a follow-up consultation with him. He said I was probably a prime contender for HRT. I was very annoyed that no one had sat down and told me about these symptoms and what might happen to me. It seemed like a typical case of medical arrogance. I had wanted someone to sit down and say to me,

'This is what you're going to have done and this is what's going to happen.'

What had happened was that my other ovary had been removed so long ago that none of the nurses had looked that far back in my notes. They hadn't realised I'd been left without any, so they didn't talk to me about it afterwards either.

I got home and thought, 'Hell, I'm having my menopause.' That threw me, it really did. It explained why I'd been very hot and red-faced and waking up at night sweating. These were all the things I remembered my mother going through.

Olivia felt very down – she thinks maybe because of the operation and the realisation that she couldn't have any more children.

Before the operation I thought, yes, it would be nice to have the option to have another one. I remember thinking that on the operating table. The surgeon said to me, 'You're lucky you've got two children.' That's what I tell myself. There are an awful lot of people out there with no children or seriously ill children. But if I'd known they might have to remove the ovary I might have frozen some eggs or something.

Olivia found HRT very helpful very quickly.

I go back and see my GP every six months or so and he checks me. I don't know how long I'll stay on it – I'm frightened to come off it and I'm only thirty-five. I felt so dreadful before I went on it. It was like a life-saver to take those tablets every day.

Olivia has an added difficulty because of her age.

> None of my contemporaries or friends have gone
> through this. They are all in a different position
> from me which wouldn't be so if my menopause
> had happened at the ordinary time.
> All I can do is put the experience behind me
> and say to myself I've got my two girls. It could
> have been worse.

If your periods seem to be slowing down and becoming
less regular this may not necessarily be a sign that your
menopause is beginning. If you're under forty, another
explanation is much more likely. Too much stress is a
common reason for periods to be missed or to become
irregular. Anorexia or any excessive weight loss is
another, as is polycystic ovarian disease – look out for the
other signs of this which include obesity and excess
bodily hair.

I would always recommend that you check with your
doctor if your period pattern changes suddenly or in a
way that puzzles or alarms you. Even if you feel one
hundred per cent sure you've reached your menopause
you may still benefit from a chat and a check-up with
your GP.

If you need to be sure you've reached the menopause
and so don't need to use contraceptives, you can either
check with your doctor, who may take a blood test, or
wait until you've had no periods for two years if you're
under fifty or one year if you're over fifty.

The menopause, as we've said, often comes at a time of
other great changes. Maybe children are leaving home,
maybe there are elderly relatives to look after, worry
about or grieve for if they've died. Maybe you or your
partner is facing a mid-life crisis – a realisation that *this* is
life, not a rehearsal as the Americans say, and a large

chunk of it's just gone. There's no doubt that levels of stress are an important factor when looking at an individual's healthy functioning and feelings of well being. If you are very stressed your symptoms will inevitably be worse and you will cope with them less well. That's another book entirely, of course, but this is always worth bearing in mind.

OSTEOPOROSIS

For many women the prospect of osteoporosis – brittle and porous bones – looms after the menopause. Estimates range between one woman in four and one woman out of every two being susceptible to this disease.

The reason the menopause is significant is that there is greater loss of bone mass when the body produces less oestrogen. A bone fracture can result from a very minor fall and this can go on to threaten life and the quality of life: half of all women who fracture a hip cannot later go on to lead an independent existence – an extraordinarily high figure. With a loss of independence can come depression and feelings of inadequacy, hopelessness and frustration – not the happiest array of emotions with which to live your last decades.

Another feature of osteoporosis is that it can develop without you realising it. It can start while you're in your thirties, without any obvious signs. Then, in later years, you might notice cupboards and shelves becoming harder to reach as you lose inches with your loss of bone density. You may also develop a 'dowager's hump' type stoop.

Other early symptoms can include back pain, which is due to crumbling vertebrae, and clothes not fitting the way they used to because your spine has started to curve. This happens when weakened bones compress then fracture and collapse. Or bones may break. Often the first sign that anything is wrong is a fractured hip or wrist after a fall. The vertebrae – the small bones that make up the spine – wrists, forearms, upper thighs and hips are most vulnerable. Men's bones are thicker and so are less vulnerable but, maybe surprisingly, one in forty men do suffer from the disease.

Osteoporosis is far from an inevitable part of growing old. As we've said, maybe only one in four women develop the disease. Until recently no one could find out whether they were likely to be included in this statistic, but now screening tests have been developed at Guy's Hospital in London which are painless and quick and which measure bone mass.

There are other indicators, however, which point to the likelihood of osteoporosis being a problem for you.

- If you had an early menopause – and late puberty.
- If there's a family history of osteoporosis – if your mother and grandmothers had the disease.
- If you didn't have children.
- If you have a small build of body – if your bones are thin and if you don't have much fat (at last there's a good, healthy reason to celebrate not being fashionably thin!).
- If you've had a low calcium diet.
- If your lifestyle's lacked exercise.
- If your diet is a high protein one.
- If your diet's low in fluoride.
- If you are or have been a heavy drinker.
- If you smoke (this slows down the production of hormones).
- If you've often used steroids.

The Office of Health Economics outlined these eleven risk factors and suggests if you have two or more you should consider taking HRT during the menopause which will help stop bone loss (of which more later).

Some experts believe this list is a better method of predicting which women are at risk than the tests which measure bone density.

The National Osteoporosis Society suggests the following may also be indicators:

- Rheumatoid arthritis, asthma and hyperparathyroidism.
- Taking certain medicines which inhibit the growth of the cells which produce bone tissue.
- Steroids taken over a long period.
- If you have a sitting-down job such as office work and take no exercise.
- If you have fair skin.
- If you drank less than a pint of milk a day as a child and adolescent.
- If your diet now does not include dairy products.
- If you've ever been confined to bed or wheelchair.
- If you've had an over-active thyroid.
- If you have scoliosis of the spine (a twisted spine).
- If you've lost height.
- If you've broken any bones other than in road traffic accidents.
- If you've always weighed under ten stone and your adult height is under five foot six.
- If you eat large helpings of uncooked bran and lots of red meat.
- If you use too many vitamin A or D supplements.
- If you use antacids made with aluminium or liquid paraffin every week.
- If your dental x-rays show periodontal disease.
- If you've used more than two months' worth of certain powerful diuretics.
- If your diet has been deficient in vitamin D (the vitamin which helps the body absorb calcium) or if

your lifestyle hasn't included a great deal of sunlight (this helps the body to produce vitamin D).
- Overtraining by athletes and dancers, which together with their restricted diet interferes with the production of hormones.

It is important that bones become denser and stronger between the ages of twenty and forty. So if you're pregnant or breastfeeding, dieting can contribute to problems and a high calcium intake is a good idea – you're feeding your baby's bones as well as your own. If you don't do this, your baby will take his or her calcium needs from your bones.

We were all taught since childhood that calcium is good for bones – and our mums were right. It's always important to have a good supply of calcium in our diet. The crucial times are during childhood, during adolescence, while pregnant, while breastfeeding and during the ten years before the menopause and the ten years afterwards when the body's absorption of calcium becomes less efficient due to hormonal changes. Cushing's Syndrome, long-term use of steroids, hyperthyroidism and alcoholism all mean less calcium for the body.

Remember, osteoporosis is thought of by many as a disease of the elderly but this is an over-simplification. Recent research among women aged fifty to fifty-four showed as many as one in three were already at risk of bone fractures from osteoporosis. Our bones may stop growing in length pretty early in our lives but there usually continues to be a build-up of bone density until about the age of thirty-five when the renewal process slows down and gradual loss of bone mass starts to occur. From thirty-five we lose more bone mass than we replace. This is less of a problem for men because they don't have the sudden drop in oestrogen levels.

It's estimated that around six thousand people a year

die prematurely because of the effects of the lack of mobility resulting from osteoporosis. In those very badly affected, annual bone loss after the menopause can be as high as 5 per cent – which would mean that roughly half of someone's bone mass will have gone within ten years of their menopause.

But less depressing news is that you can have osteoporosis for years without knowing it. Some women, even fifteen years after the menopause, aren't in any pain. Also it used to be thought that osteoporosis was irreversible; however recent studies suggest that among women taking HRT some bone density is replaced.

Chris

Nursing on an orthopaedic ward gave Chris two reasons to take HRT. First, the amount of lifting of heavy bodies she had to do meant she had to have a cartilage removed from her knee. After her operation it seemed as if her menopause had been triggered as she started to get hot flushes and sweats.

> They were really bad. My night sweats meant I had to get up at least twice in the night to change my nightie. I'd have to move and sleep in the spare bedroom because my side of the bed would be soaking wet.

The other reason was the number of women she'd nursed with terrible osteoporotic fractures. She knew she didn't want that to be her. Ever.

> Lifting those dear old things with their broken hips and wrists and humped shoulders had a big effect on me. I'd grab hold of their daughters and daughters-in-law when they were visiting and say, 'Have you heard of HRT?'

A lot of seventy- and eighty-year-olds who came in never got home again. The shock of the fall they'd had was too much for them. It would be absolutely traumatic and would really confuse them.

If you fall or nearly fall it makes you quiver inside – you catch your breath. But when you're slightly unsure on your feet anyway, you're getting old and you've got a bit of arthritis and you fall and break something you can get confused. The anaesthetic can affect you too. And being confined to bed makes your blood more likely to clot, perhaps resulting in all kinds of potentially life-threatening problems.

Chris remembers trying to coax her patients to walk after their hips had been replaced.

They don't want to. They're petrified. They will cling to you. They're frightened because they think they'll fall again. You're there, they have a zimmer frame and a physio giving exercises to build up their confidence, and they're still frightened. Sometimes they've spent all their lives in their own home and have coped marvellously. Now they can't cope when they get home because of their fall. Then that puts an added strain on the family who have the mother or mother-in-law staying with them or sometimes they have to go into a home, which is so traumatic and upsetting for them.

Now fifty-two, Chris has been on HRT for five years and as well as the long-term protection she wants against osteoporosis, it's made a big difference to her life.

I have a wonderful, understanding husband but I became so irritable during the menopause I was flying off the handle at the slightest thing. I could feel myself do it but there was nothing I could do to stop myself. It was like having terrible, terrible PMT and it would happen at any time.

I wouldn't do the housework and then in the last hour before I had to leave for work I'd try to do it all – hoover, do the washing, everything. It was very, very stressful. I'd never want to go into work and when I went in that would be stressful because it was understaffed and one day I just cracked up. I rang up my supervisor and said I was at my wits' end. She sent me an extra nurse but normally I could have coped without. I felt terrible for making the fuss. That's when I decided I had to go to see my GP.

This had all happened while Chris had been taking a form of Hormone Replacement. She went to her doctor to get her prescription changed but found she wasn't sympathetic at all, merely upping the dosage of the pills. 'They were worse. I had headaches and felt ill,' Chris remembers.

My husband had been in a book shop and he'd seen a book about the Amarant Centre which promotes HRT and told me he thought I'd find it interesting because the women in the book seemed to be going through the same sort of thing. I bought it and read it and thought, 'This sounds like me.'

I asked my doctor to refer me to the Amarant Centre because we weren't getting anywhere and when they said, 'Of course we can help you,' it was such a relief.

Chris is sure it saved her marriage.

> My husband was coming home from work and
> the moment he walked through the door I'd let
> rip at him about all these things I'd saved up all
> day to throw at him when I saw him. We'd have
> blazing rows. He said, 'I only come home to walk
> the dog. If it hadn't been for the dog I'd have left
> long ago.' I'd also have rows with my two sons –
> terrible up and downers. I could never see their
> point of view. I was always right. We'd row about
> the length of their hair – anything. There was an
> awful atmosphere in the house.
>
> Looking back now I wasn't behaving properly
> but I couldn't have done anything about it. It was
> like there was a barrier but I couldn't climb over
> it or get through it to behave normally.

Chris had also started getting problems with her
breasts, which became hard and lumpy. So she was
relieved when the Amarant Centre put her on a different
type of HRT. Since then she's had to have a hysterectomy
for other reasons and now has the hormone replacement
patch which she says is marvellous. 'I don't have any
problems at all although there are odd days when I'm
grumpy and grouchy,' she admits.

Recently Chris's mother has had to move into warden-
controlled flats after an accident – instead of using her
small step-ladder to reach a high cupboard she used a
stool because it would be quicker, slipped, fell and broke
her wrist, probably a result of osteoporosis. 'She is happy
there now although she wasn't at first,' says Chris. 'It just
showed me how precarious life can be. I know if we can
prevent osteoporosis we will go into our seventies and
eighties so much fitter and more independent.'

HEART ATTACKS AND STROKES

Before the menopause a woman's risk of heart disease is only a fifth of that of a man. But, after the menopause, the statistical sex difference disappears as her oestrogen levels fall. This leaves heart attacks as the most frequent cause of death in women, with strokes as the second most frequent cause. A very different picture.

Heart attacks can be the result of one of two main problems. The first is that the coronary arteries which carry the blood supply to the heart muscle are hindered in their work by a build-up of fatty substances on their walls. The second is a thrombosis, which means a clot forms in the coronary artery. If this clot develops where the artery has narrowed, the blood supply to the heart muscle will be cut off and a heart attack will be the result.

According to a study by the Medical Research Council, HRT users are only half as likely to die from heart attacks or strokes as women not taking the therapy. Oestrogen is known to reduce the development of clogged arteries and is good for the blood vessels, improving the cardio-vascular system overall.

There have been worries that the protection given through taking oestrogen might be countered by the progestogen added to most preparations for the latter part of each month. This is no longer thought to be the case although the protection probably isn't quite as great as that provided by oestrogen alone.

But are you likely to be at risk from a heart attack after your menopause? The British Heart Foundation suggests these are likely indicators that you might be:

- If either of your parents or a brother or sister had a heart attack, particularly under the age of fifty-five for female relatives and fifty for male relatives.
- If you have ever smoked – especially if it was in the recent past or you are still smoking. Stopping smoking

is by far the best action you can take (and it lessens the chance of lung cancer as well). If you smoke and are taking the contraceptive pill this is particularly dangerous.

- If you are overweight (a very fatty diet, especially, will raise your cholesterol level). In the United Kingdom, 12 per cent of women, that's one in eight, are 'obese' – very overweight indeed.
- If you do very little exercise – and physical activity often declines with age. It was recently revealed that the level of physical activity carried out by eight out of ten women is below that needed for cardiovascular health.
- If you have raised blood pressure (your doctor will check this for you).
- If you have a raised blood cholesterol level (your doctor will tell you if he considers a test necessary – they're not recommended to everyone, especially people who do not come from families where high cholesterol levels are a problem). Cholesterol levels rise with age and by fifty-five more than three-quarters of women have levels above that recommended.
- If you suffer from diabetes.
- If you are very stressed. (This association with heart attacks is less certain especially for initial heart attacks. It is thought more likely to be a risk factor where there is existing heart disease.)

   The exception to this is if your stress shows itself in the form of panic attacks – women who have panic attacks and hyperventilate sometimes get coronary artery spasms. Eighty per cent of people who have panic attacks are women and up to 14 per cent of patients seeing heart specialists have these panic disorders.

- There's a suggestion that drugs for depression and anxiety might make heart attacks more likely – but on the other hand if they weren't taken panic attacks might be more likely, so giving them up and panicking might not be a good idea.

The Foundation stresses that the degree to which you are at risk depends on a combination of all these factors – so if you have slightly raised blood pressure it's not necessarily the end of the road for you. Your risk may be no more than average if you pass our checklist in most of the other categories. They suggest this is especially true of slightly or moderately raised cholesterol levels – if you don't smoke and your blood pressure is normal, this isn't worth losing sleep about. And they emphasise that even if you've a higher than average risk of a coronary, the chances are even greater that you won't have one.

Of course even if you followed all the rules – lost weight, packed in smoking, leapt into your local swimming pool on a regular basis – there's no absolute guarantee of preventing heart disease, but doing these things will reduce your risk and make you feel healthier and livelier.

Judith

With close members of both sides of her family suffering from heart disease, Judith knew she was a high risk. 'I am concerned about that – especially as I have a sit-down job and I never exercise.' It's one of the reasons she decided to take Hormone Replacement Therapy during the menopause, despite the scare stories about breast cancer she noticed at the time. 'There has never been any breast cancer in my family so if that's a risk I'll take it,' she says. 'And if I keep an eye on it and get myself checked, I won't worry about it.'

Judith has had an on-off relationship with HRT. She started on it when, about four years ago, she would find herself crying in the street.

It would just happen. I'd be afraid to cross roads as well. I'd look both ways several times and still falter. I was also unsure of myself driving a car. I really wondered if I was going crazy.

Her periods had stopped and she thought these might be menopausal symptoms. She felt sure this was so when she began having big, angry mood swings.

I started taking HRT, but then I found myself with really heavy periods and terrible PMT. I thought my periods were behind me and wasn't wanting this at all. I thought, 'This is it. I'm going to stop.'
I came off and for a month it was great. I thought, 'Who needs it?'

Her response came swiftly.

At fifty-four all of a sudden I found myself with all these menopausal symptoms. Every one you can think of. I had terrible sweats. I began to look older. My skin turned greyish – except when I had hot flushes that is! I didn't realise it would be this extreme. I went back to my GP and told him I felt I was caught between the devil and the deep blue sea. Either I would have horrible periods and PMT cramps or this. He offered me a new prescription which I wouldn't take.

Instead, like Chris, Judith went to the Amarant Centre.

It turned out they too gave me the one my doctor was offering me. I couldn't believe my doctor had got it right! I'm taking the brand which means you don't get bleeding – it's called Livial [see page 48].

I'm very happy with it now although I have put on a bit of weight. And I'm especially pleased because I know of the protection it offers my heart. I feel I'm protecting my present and my future.

THE 'MALE MENOPAUSE'

The male menopause is a less cut and dried affair than that of the female. There's no sudden fall off in hormone levels as there is during a woman's menopause. For many the term 'mid-life crisis' seems more appropriate when talking about what it is that men experience.

Having said this, some of the symptoms men complain of are surprisingly similar to those of women during the same time. Men have suffered hot flushes and sweating and, more commonly, depression, fatigue, loss of sexual interest and drive, and aches and pains. One specialist treats these symptoms with testosterone and says the male menopause – which he calls the viropause – usually affects highly stressed, unfit businessmen, who drink and maybe eat too much, as well as men who've had mumps or vasectomies. The unproven theory behind this is that all these activities and events diminish the man's natural production of testosterone.

However other more conventional experts say any male menopause observed is not hormonal and treating with testosterone could be hazardous, leading to heart disease, prostate or liver problems. This second view is the prevalent one, but how will we persuade men – who are maybe seeing their wives' renewed energy and interest in sex and want some of 'whatever they're having' – of this? Indeed, some of the partners of women on HRT have found it a problem that they haven't the stamina to match their wives!

Chapter Two
HORMONE REPLACEMENT THERAPY

One in ten women in Britain of menopausal age are taking or have taken Hormone Replacement Therapy and it's becoming increasingly popular – although still less so than in America, France and other countries in Europe.

Many specialists think it will be prescribed routinely in the future, such is its success as a preventative medicine. But, having said that, it's clear that around 20 per cent of women don't need it anyway. These are the women who continue to produce oestrogen – albeit 'weak' oestrogen – during and after their menopause, a substance called oestrone. This is most likely to occur in women who are slightly overweight (another good reason not to be fashionably pencil thin).

It is clear from Mike's postbag that it's not just the long-term health benefits which attract women to HRT. Countless times he's learned of the relief felt as hot flushes, mood swings and night sweats disappear. The emotional stress which women feel, resulting from the effect of the menopause on their emotional stability, is lifted. Relationships become happier and more harmonious. In fact, in our experience, it is often for these reasons rather than for the long-term health benefits that women want HRT.

Another plus factor for HRT is that it's suitable for nearly all women and can often take effect very quickly – even as fast as a couple of weeks after you start taking it.

The *Daily Express* survey from a couple of years ago reported 90 per cent of women taking HRT as saying it improved their health, including 20 per cent who said their symptoms had completely disappeared. A third said their libido had increased and they felt they looked better – their skin and shape had improved. They also found they coped better both at work and at home.

What they said, and what seems to be almost universally true for women who try HRT, is that if you're having a difficult menopause and you decide to take HRT for a few years you will probably sail through it.

The HRT supporters, who believe the positive effects of HRT are so great they'd like to see all women given the therapy for ten years, have a lot of persuasive arguments on their side. Researchers are finding that when women stop having periods their risk of heart disease rises to that of men. Before this, as we've already mentioned, it's much lower. HRT could bring those levels down again by up to 50 per cent. But, having said that, not everyone is at risk from heart disease.

When it comes to bones, HRT protects against calcium loss. For maximum bone protection, you should start taking HRT within five years of starting your menopause. The treatment will then prevent bone loss, but only while it is taken. Similarly, if your bone loss is already a problem, while taken HRT will halt the decline in your bone density.

Certain types of arthritis, where osteoporosis interferes with the structure or normal working of the joints, are less likely if you are taking HRT. Arthritis of the spine, for example, like cervical spondylosis, is made much worse by osteoporosis.

Another less well-known positive effect of HRT is its treatment of incontinence. It's thought around one in three women suffer this distressing and embarrassing condition after their menopause. In some cases hormone replacement will help – especially if your incontinence is of the form known as 'sudden urge incontinence', due to an over-sensitive bladder-triggering mechanism, rather than leakage which comes after a sneeze or other sudden similar stress.

There are also suggestions that HRT can save you from the general degeneration that comes with age – though we think that may be stretching it a bit.

Some women, it has to be admitted, take HRT in the hope that it will help them keep their looks and their vitality in the future. Doctors do not usually prescribe on that basis, however. HRT is prescribed for medical reasons, such as to encourage vaginal secretions and to keep bones strong, not to preserve glamour. But you don't need to be a medical expert to know that looking good and feeling good are so often interlinked.

Many women find they have unpleasant side-effects from taking HRT. We'll go into more detail about these at the end of this chapter, but they can include mood swings, which are sometimes very intense, tenderness of breasts, cramps, nausea, depression, bloatedness and weight gain caused mostly by the progestogen element if it is HRT composed of the combined hormones. However, it's not that simple. For every individual you do need to have exactly the right medication or dose for you, to keep side-effects to a minimum.

Another possible side-effect is the despondency which can come from raised expectations of HRT. In a way it is a victim of its own success. Many women read the astonishing reports of its effectiveness and expect a wonder drug which they may then find isn't so wonderful for them. Sometimes a change of prescription is the answer or a change of dose; sometimes women carry on taking the HRT despite the side-effects, and sometimes, in time, the side-effects disappear.

The side-effect that's most commonly complained about is the continuation of monthly bleeding. This doesn't happen with all HRT. If you have had a hysterectomy you will have an oestrogen-only form which won't cause 'periods'. But if you haven't you will probably be prescribed a combined oestrogen and progestogen form as oestrogen on its own could cause cancer of the womb lining. A low dose of progestogen prescribed with the oestrogen and taken for ten or twelve consecutive days at the end of each protects against womb cancer. However the progestogen causes the womb to shed its lining in a regular bleed, similar to a light period, and you'll need to use tampons or sanitary towels. Some women worry that these bleeds mean that fertility has returned and that they may become pregnant, but this fear is quite unfounded. A new development might mean an end to bleeding with the combined HRT but more of that later (see page 48).

Another concern is that HRT may increase the risk of breast cancer. The evidence for this is conflicting. One Swedish study showed an increased risk but this used a strong synthetic type of oestrogen that is not used here. Specialists in the UK where the 'weaker' natural oestrogens are used say there's no increased risk if you take this natural type of HRT for up to six years and probably none if you take it for up to ten years. After ten years there is probably a small increase in the risk of breast cancer but no increase in deaths caused by it. This may be because of the extra care taken by women on HRT both to check themselves and to get checked so any problems are hopefully found and dealt with earlier.

However, it's true that with breast cancer even a small increased risk is significant because this cancer is a widespread disease.

There is no known link between HRT and cervical cancer. The scares began in the 1970s when the risk of cancer of the lining of the womb was linked to women taking oestrogen-only HRT. Then progestogen was added and the risk was removed. In fact, there's then less risk of womb cancer than among those not taking HRT at all. However, the need for progestogen to be given as well is on the grounds of caution and this is wise although the risk without it is very small.

Having said all this, some women have been taking HRT for twenty years or more with no ill-effects and a happier, healthier lifestyle to show for it. They may be taking more of a risk but those risks are still small. Amazingly, in the United States, doctors are actually being sued for failing to mention HRT and its benefits to their patients.

But the miracles some women are expecting won't materialise. Most importantly HRT won't keep you young. It won't stop you from ageing – although it will increase the collagen content of the skin and help it to retain water which disguises wrinkles and lines. This is one of the objections some of HRT's opponents have to it. They include Germaine Greer who recently wrote in her book *The Change: Women, Ageing and the Menopause*, 'A grown woman should not have to masquerade as a girl in order to remain in the land of the living.' True, very true. But our culture, which so promotes the beauty of the young and youthful over the beauty of experience and maturity, is very deeply instilled in all of us, men and women alike.

More warning bells are rung by those who suggest that oestrogen is such a plus for women – lifting their mood and making them feel so good – that they don't want to stop taking it. The claim is that women can become emotionally dependent on HRT, maybe thinking they won't be attractive or desirable without it. Giving up HRT would be like giving up their protection against ageing, whatever the consequences for their health. On the same lines, there are suggestions of physical dependency on HRT – which would mostly affect women who had increased their dose to get more effect and who would then find they were experiencing withdrawal symptoms when they tried to stop taking it. Apparently when implants of HRT aren't available some women increase their oral or patch dose, perhaps wearing several patches at once. They feel cravings and find themselves depressed and tired if their dosage is lowered.

How much of this is true and how much sensationalism, it's difficult to say. But what's clear is that it's vital women do not take it upon themselves to increase their dosage. If you feel you need a higher dose then ask your doctor what he or she thinks. If you're depressed for reasons which are nothing to do with losing out on oestrogen then more and more HRT won't help you fight your depression. It might land you with another problem instead.

While we're on the subject of opposition, there's a claim from another opponent of HRT, Dr Ellen Grant, author of *The Bitter Pill*, that's staggering. She says surveys show that women who have taken HRT for at least a year are two and a half times more likely to commit or attempt to commit suicide. She explains this by suggesting that oestrogen can block the body's metabolism of common anti-depressants, increasing their toxic side-effects. She also claims that the hormones used in HRT are harmful even though they are naturally produced, unlike the artificial ones used in the manufacture of the contraceptive pill. She also claims there is more ovarian cancer among HRT takers, and suggests that the cardiovascular benefits might be the result of the way those who take HRT are selected – women using the therapy are more likely to be non-smokers, for example.

Even though we've looked at her ideas with interest, we see no reason to adjust our position. Of course there are risks but we feel the benefits are much stronger than she has suggested. It's always a question of balancing the advantages and the risks. If you're considering taking

HRT you may be reassured by figures quoted by a spokesman for the Menopause Society which show that of 100,000 women taking HRT for fifteen years, at worst 187 more would die of breast cancer, but deaths from heart disease would be down by 5250 and deaths from a fractured hip down by 563.

It's very important that you take the therapy for a few years so that your body does benefit from it, although a lot of women do give up more quickly, mainly because they don't like having monthly bleeds which usually come with the joint oestrogen and progestogen HRT.

If you're taking it to protect against osteoporosis and cardiovascular diseases then it needs to be taken for a much longer period of time still. This allows calcium to be absorbed more efficiently, stops bone loss and has a positive effect on the heart.

WHEN TO SEEK HELP

It is quite a good idea to visit your doctor at the first signs of the menopause, as this is an ideal time for a check-up and a check-over. Make a note of any symptoms you've had, when your last period was and what, if anything, happened that was different.

If you're interested in Hormone Replacement Therapy this is usually the time you might expect to be given your first prescription. When you have to wait seven or eight weeks between periods or when you've missed three HRT could start being useful. There's no point in getting a head-start with HRT. I know some women are so keen to avoid troublesome symptoms, or serious illness later in life, they want to start 'yesterday', but that's not advisable even if it were possible. If you start too early you could get side-effects as you'll be upsetting your body's natural balance of oestrogen. You might get irregular bleeding and may need to be referred for a D&C or a uterine-lining biopsy. Not a lot of fun!

So wait until you have your first menopausal symptoms or your periods stop – an indication that you've started not to produce your full quota of hormones.

Something else to bear in mind is that you might jump the gun inadvertently. You may have a couple of hot flushes and assume your menopause is starting and it's time for HRT, but many women in their forties have flushes as a symptom of Pre-Menstrual Syndrome and they may carry on having periods for years and years after their flushes begin. It is usual to start HRT at forty-five or older.

The symptoms to look out for to be more or less sure you're entering your menopause are irregular periods or no periods at all, night sweats and hot flushes.

Jean

Jean, a part-time secretary, was in no doubt what she would do when her menopause began.

> I've got friends who are five or ten years older than me and they all take HRT. And with my first flush I was down at the doctor's. I had no intention of suffering from any of the things they had told me about or I had read about in magazines.

She found her doctor was against HRT – she thinks he was concerned about the publicity surrounding cancer risks – and he wouldn't prescribe it for her. Instead he prescribed a medicine to relieve her physical symptoms which only worked for a short time.

> After that he still refused me HRT so I went to

my local chemist and asked her if she'd noticed on the prescriptions she handed out which local doctors were in favour of hormone replacement.

The chemist gave her the information and Jean changed her doctor.

I was most scared about the possibility of getting depressed. Friends of mine had talked about how they'd go round their homes wringing their hands with worry and I knew I didn't want any of that. Especially when the other drugs he gave me didn't stop the hot flushes, I was determined to get HRT.

Jean, who's fifty-four, has now been receiving hormone replacement treatment for five years and is so far the only one in her family to take HRT.

My mother says she didn't have a very difficult menopause. She 'worked' her way through it – she got by without any help from anyone. My youngest sister hasn't started hers yet and my other sister says she's prepared to work her way through hers as well. I think she's worried about possible side-effects.

But if my doctor takes me off it I will look for another doctor. I don't see any reason not to take it – I certainly don't want to get a humpy back.

I remember seeing Kate O'Mara, the actress on television, saying it gave her a new lease of life and I thought, 'Why not me as well?' I've carried on exactly as I was before the menopause.

Jean had made her mind up and is obviously happy with the treatment she's getting. But do remember that not every woman suffers severe symptoms and for some women the menopause really is trouble-free.

Another point that's worth remembering is that you won't miss your moment if you don't turn up on your GP's doorstep when your symptoms first begin. If you want to see if you can cope without medication, that's fine – it's never too late for you to seek advice. Help is at hand even if your last period is long gone. For example, vaginal dryness and pain on urinating and intercourse, can certainly be rectified despite the time lapse. Mike remembers receiving a letter from a sixty-year-old woman who'd never married, indeed who'd never had sexual intercourse, and who suddenly found a 'boyfriend' ten years after her menopause. Vaginal dryness, until then, hadn't been important or a problem. HRT or an oestrogen cream would have been a solution. Mike was able to persuade her to overcome her embarrassment and consult her doctor and the newer HRT, Livial, was prescribed – which meant she was spared the monthly 'period'. Unfortunately in order to stop osteoporosis developing you do need to start taking HRT within five years of your menopause, although starting later can halt the process and may recover some of the lost bone.

The response of Jean's doctor isn't that unusual, we have to say. It is frightening for doctors as well as for patients to learn of possible breast cancer risks and this may be enough to make them shy away from prescribing HRT. However this view is becoming less and less common. All of the positive publicity HRT has received and the obvious positive effects it's had on women have led to a change in attitude. As far as we're concerned, if a woman is getting symptoms which are unpleasant and undermining and she's suffering unnecessarily, why not suggest HRT?

In our opinion the reason most women want HRT is

because of the discomfort and embarrassment of hot flushes and night sweats and the grim feelings which surround depression and moodiness rather than wanting to invest in protection for their bones and heart. However, like Jean, once on the medication they are likely to become aware of the other health benefits HRT can offer and they too can be very tempting.

The immediate symptoms can be serious enough in themselves.Hot flushes may not last long – or they may last for ten years or more. You may spend your time wanting to strangle your son or daughter or your dog or cat or husband or neighbour. You may be aware of the negative effect your mood is having on your relationships and see no way out of this. None of this is going to help you like yourself very much.

HRT should also be advised if you have lost your ovaries from surgery or through radiation treatment or if you've had a hysterectomy. If you don't have a womb, you can have the oestrogen-only type of HRT which means you will miss out on a lot of the potential side-effects which progestogen might cause. However only a small percentage of women who've had hysterectomies are prescribed HRT. Without it they can face a greater loss of sex drive and a greater risk of heart attack and osteoporosis, especially if hysterectomy together with the removal of the ovaries took place when they were relatively young.

Health checks should be available to you before and while you take HRT. Before you begin the therapy, some doctors suggest that a blood test, a mammogram and similar tests are carried out to see that you are in normal health. Many, if not most others, think that a chat and maybe a physical examination and blood pressure check is just as good and far less fuss and expense.

Earlier in this book we've mentioned the possibility of getting a bone scan to see if you might be susceptible to osteoporosis. This can be carried out by sophisticated machinery in leading hospitals which measures the bone density of your spine and hip. It can register bone loss at a very early stage and looks at bone density in the places where osteoporosis is most likely to be found. If you have a series of scans you can see how fast your bone loss is. However this equipment is not available to all because, as far as we know, it can only be found in twenty National Health Service hospitals, far fewer than could meet the demand. It's not a technique which is generally thought to be essential for all, so private tests may, unfortunately, be the only option if you can afford it and when it's considered to be a good idea.

Your doctor might suggest other alternatives to HRT. You may be offered tranquillisers if you are feeling stressed, anti-depressants if you are feeling depressed, or counselling if you are both of these.

Tranquillisers have a bad name but do have a short-term use, we believe, at periods of very heavy stress by calming anxiety and relieving sleeplessness. However they do not solve any problems or worries you may have, simply anaesthetise them for a short time. If you do not want to try HRT but do feel at the end of your tether this might be a short-term option. Remember, tranquillisers are addictive, so we do stress 'short-term'.

Anti-depressants aren't addictive and they can relieve deep feelings of depression and remove some physical symptoms to help the sufferer cope with life more easily.

Counselling is a more time-consuming and more challenging option which involves looking at the root causes of your bad feelings. If you're feeling unloved and uncared for because your children are staying out late all the time or leaving home, if you're feeling in a rut with your partner and that your life has passed you by, if you're dreading old age and loneliness and can think of nothing exciting to anticipate in the years to come, maybe your mood isn't simply hormone-related, or isn't hormone-related at all. You may have deep-seated feelings which you could discuss with a counsellor. Doing so really can be a great relief.

Some counsellors may be seen free on the NHS – some medical practices have counsellors linked to them – or you may find one through the organisations listed at the end of the book. Most you have to pay for but sometimes they are open-minded about this if you don't have the cash.

You can see a counsellor for short-term problems – and remember the counsellor is not there to judge you but to listen genuinely and empathetically. Psychotherapy involves looking at longer-term problems more intensively and here you will do most of the talking yourself. Psychoanalysis concentrates on looking at your dreams and childhood, at both your conscious and unconscious life and, if not an answer to short-term problems, it may have long-term benefits. Not every counsellor is suitable for every client so you may have to try one or two before you find one who suits you. Once you've done this it can be a great relief to talk to someone knowledgeable and understanding and to know this is time just for you.

Pamela

Pamela's symptoms were not the usual ones although they will be recognised by many women, we're sure. There were no hot flushes or night sweats. Her symptoms were far more difficult to pin down.

> I was getting anxiety attacks and forgetting names. I was continually having to take time off work since I felt unsafe when I was away from home – a bit like a phobia that a friend of mine had really. It completely upset my routine, I went off my food and I couldn't sleep properly. I felt my

world was falling apart. I had previously asked my GP about HRT and asked whether this would help, as it seemed to me that this was something I hadn't experienced before and I read somewhere that unusual happenings at the time of the menopause could be due to that. My GP hadn't been in favour.

But when in desperation I returned to see my doctor he was on holiday and I had to see his partner. He said that I hadn't much to lose by trying HRT and that's what was decided.

Once I went on it the panic went – almost immediately. I haven't looked back since then and I now feel very calm and able to cope.

WHAT'S AVAILABLE?

There are two main types of Hormone Replacement Therapy:

- Oestrogen only – for women who have had a hysterectomy. This is because research suggests that oestrogen by itself can increase the risk of cancer of the womb lining – the endometrium. If you have had your womb removed in a hysterectomy you no longer have a womb lining.
- Oestrogen and progestogen. Progestogen is added half way through each cycle and taken for 10–12 days because it neutralises oestrogen's capacity to create womb-lining cancer by removing the lining in the form of a period. Unlike those used in the contraceptive Pill which are manufactured, some oestrogens used in Hormone Replacement Therapy include natural oestrogen produced from animal sources as well as manufactured ones which act like natural hormones.

There are different methods of taking HRT – different routes are right for different women. See table on p. 99.

1. The daily tablet. These are small pill-sized tablets, with oestrogen and progestogen taken in sequence, or oestrogen taken on its own. Because these are taken by mouth the oestrogen passes through the liver before circulating to the rest of the body. This means that the dose needs to be higher because some of the oestrogen is broken down in the liver before it is distributed around the body rather than reaching the body by a more direct route. If you are taking both oestrogen and progestogen you take the oestrogen pill alone for the first half of the cycle, then add the progestogen for the last ten, or twelve days depending on the type prescribed. You may start the twenty-eight-day cycle again without a break or have seven pill-free days, depending again on the type prescribed. We recommend the twelve-day progestogen regime, since it gives the best possible womb-lining protection. The most commonly prescribed combined regimes are Prempak C and Cyclo-Progynova.

The HRT pill has been around for decades and is the most popular method for taking HRT at present.

2. Implants. With this system, a pellet about the size of an apple pip is implanted into a woman's body in a couple of minutes under a local anaesthetic, in the doctor's surgery. The implant lasts for up to six months. In addition, if you haven't had a hysterectomy, you would also need to take a progestogen pill for twelve days of each monthly cycle. When menopausal symptoms come back a new implant is given.

One suggested disadvantage of this system is the possibility that the implant can produce tachyphylaxis – the need to increase the dose each time to get the same effect. Specialist opinion differs as to whether this is correct. Another disadvantage is that some women say they need more and more regular implants to feel the same – the hormones seem to be getting used up more quickly than expected and levels in the bloodstream may be variable. Another disadvantage is that you need 'surgery' – i.e. an implant injection – about every six months. Also, if the implant has to be removed for whatever reason, this can be very difficult to achieve. But the good side of using implants is that it means you don't have to remember to pop pills or change patches.

3. Patches. This is the newest method. You stick a patch which looks like clear plastic sticking plaster and is slightly bigger than a 50p piece on to your buttock. You change the patch twice a week and, if you haven't had a hysterectomy, you also take a progestogen pill for twelve days a month. The hormone oestrogen reaches the bloodstream by passing through the skin, thus avoiding the liver, and this is thought to be better. This method also means that smaller quantities of hormones are needed. The oestrogen patch is called Estraderm and can also be prescribed to include 12 progestogen pills when it is known as Estrapak.

Recently a new patch has become available which includes both oestrogen and progestogen. The makers of Estracombi – its trade name – claim adverse effects are less likely than when pills are used and so, hopefully, there will be fewer problems such as bloating and sore breasts. Another advantage of this is that some users of patches had been intentionally missing out on taking their progestogen tablets because they didn't like the side-effects they were getting and by doing this they could be increasing their risk of womb cancer. As the side-effects either don't occur or aren't as troublesome with Estracombi, they should be more encouraged to follow the correct instruction.

You still need to change the Estracombi patch twice a week but for two weeks you use oestrogen-only patches and for two weeks a double patch of oestrogen and progestogen.

4. Vaginal creams and pessaries. A low-dose vaginal cream can be prescribed specifically to relieve vaginal dryness and urinary problems. It is usually very helpful, particularly for older women well past the menopause. However, it does not provide the other benefits of HRT. For women who suffer unpleasant side-effects from HRT in the form of pills or patches, higher dose vaginal creams or pessaries are occasionally prescribed, along with progestogen tablets for those who still have a womb. A potential disadvantage of the higher dose is that some oestrogen is likely to be absorbed by the woman's partner during intercourse.

Mike often receives letters from his readers and listeners saying they're worried about changing their pills to patches although that's what their doctors have recommended. Husbands, too, having become used to the benefits that HRT has given their wives, are sometimes frightened that mood swings and depression might return. The main worry of all concerned is that the patch won't be as effective as the pills.

Of course there are bound to be worries if you are being advised to alter something that has brought you, and your family, tremendous relief. It's very easy for doctors to suggest a change and less easy for patients to understand the pros and cons of something new.

But the patch does have many advantages – and not only that smaller quantities of oestrogen are needed for the same effect. Another is that the level of hormones released into the body is kept steady because the patch releases them in a controlled way. If you're using pills, the oestrogen concentration fluctuates up and down each day, the level being determined by how long it's been since you took the last dose.

These fluctuations are another reason for the pills having a larger amount of the hormone in them, in order to keep a satisfactory level of oestrogen in the body throughout the twenty-four hours until the next pill is taken. And it really is true that, as a general rule, it's always better to use the least amount of medication necessary to achieve the desired effect.

The answer then to those letters is that there needn't be any worries about the effectiveness of the patch as it's been found to be at least as beneficial as the pill.

The patch will usually even stay on if you're going swimming or having a bath or shower as the adhesive is very strong. But many women prefer to remove the plaster before going into the water and then to replace it afterwards. We recommend this method. You don't lose the patch that way and it makes no difference to the benefits.

However there's another interesting new development. Many women stop taking HRT because they dislike the fact that they continue to have a monthly bleed when they felt they had put their periods behind them. But now there's a new HRT pill with the brand name Livial which uses a completely different hormone. This hormone doesn't cause a build-up of the womb lining which means the added progestogens aren't necessary. Because of this, monthly bleeds are avoided. Studies have shown that Livial is just as effective as oestrogen for menopausal symptoms such as hot flushes, sweating, depression and loss of libido and appears to prevent, and may even treat, osteoporosis. Livial's manufacturers recommend that it's not started until at least a year after a woman's periods have stopped as by then most women's natural oestrogen hormone production will have ceased and therefore the lining of her womb will have settled down. A very few women will have slight spotting in the initial months of taking Livial but this normally soon stops.

HOW TO HANDLE YOUR DOCTOR

Most doctors have strong attitudes towards HRT. Of course they are there to give you the treatment you need but their views on that will be influenced by their personal preferences. So it's important you play your part in deciding what is right for you and what you expect you will be happy with.

Angela

Angela's doctor was not in favour of HRT and he prescribed her anti-depressants to combat her symptoms.

I was depressed and I'd lost my confidence completely. I'd be frightened to go out. I'd cry at anything and I couldn't sleep. I also had hot flushes.

I was working on a market stall at the time and I really liked my job but because I couldn't face people I couldn't do it. Sometimes I just couldn't face going to work. I really was becoming a wreck.

I wanted to be alone. I didn't want to talk to people. I wanted to take HRT because I had a feeling it would help but my doctor isn't a believer. Instead he put me on anti-depressants but they made me feel worse. I went back to him and I told him I wanted HRT and he wrote me a prescription for different anti-depressants. I told

> him I wouldn't take them and eventually he
> wrote me a prescription for HRT.

After two or three weeks on HRT she felt a lot better.
After a year on them, and feeling fine with them, her
doctor suggested she'd been on them long enough and
she was weaned off them. Now her hot flushes are
coming back and she's hoping to start HRT again.

> I never want to get as bad as I felt then. Even if
> my symptoms don't get any worse than they are
> now I want to go back on it. HRT really helped
> me.

Angela sounds like someone who knows how to get what
she wants. You have a right to know the drawbacks and
advantages of each individual method of treating your
menopausal symptoms. A piece of paper in your hand is
not enough if you have questions you want answered
and feelings you wish to express. Likewise, your doctor
has to recommend treatment based on his knowledge
and experience so tell your doctor what your symptoms
are – maybe keeping a note of them in a kind of symptoms
diary as they occur might be useful.

Don't just stick to the physical symptoms if you have
emotional symptoms as well. Your doctor will want to
know if menopausal problems are affecting your home
life and working life and your relationships generally. Tell
him what your worries for the future are, and whether
you have osteoporosis or cardiovascular disease in the
family, perhaps.

Try not to be too embarrassed to talk to your doctor
about intimate information such as the effect of your
menopause on your sexual life. If you feel you can't talk
to him or her and you do have specific problems, say with
vaginal dryness, then changing your doctor might be an

option you could consider. Remember, whatever you're about to tell your GP, it's almost undoubtedly true that he or she will have heard it before from someone else. Your doctor isn't there to judge you but to use all the information he or she can gain to help you solve your medical problem.

If possible it's a good idea to make an appointment at a time when your doctor might be less busy. Take any notes you've jotted down with you in case you feel a bit nervous or rushed once you're there. This will also help you get your information over in a short, concise way which will be useful to your doctor. If you decide not to tell your GP about things that are really worrying you, you will be left with those anxieties when your visit is over. You may be worried that they will sound trivial but you are spending your time visiting the person who may be able to put your mind at rest or who may feel further investigations are necessary.

We have both heard complaints from countless women that their doctors – men and women – sometimes appear to show little interest in hearing about menopausal problems. That they feel belittled by their doctor's attitude. We feel that when you leave a doctor's surgery you should walk away with a feeling of being taken seriously and listened to. If you have lost confidence in your doctor it will be difficult, if not impossible, for the two of you to have a good working relationship.

We spotted a survey recently which gives some indication of what women found when they went to their doctors with menopausal complaints. In round numbers these came to:

- 12 per cent of doctors were sympathetic and prescribed tranquillisers
- 41 per cent were sympathetic and prescribed HRT

- 23 per cent were sympathetic and gave advice but no prescription
- 9 per cent were unsympathetic and unhelpful
- 7 per cent were unsympathetic and prescribed HRT
- 13 per cent referred their patients to a specialist

If this is true, that's not too bad a picture, but of course there is room for improvement. The survey also indicates that if you're not happy, doctors sympathetic to menopausal problems do exist and you'll be very unlucky, unless you live in a remote area, if there isn't one near you.

WHO CANNOT TAKE HRT?

HRT isn't suitable for everyone and it's vital your doctor is aware of your full medical history before prescribing. It's not suitable for a woman who has had recent breast cancer, severe jaundice, some forms of thrombosis, womb-lining cancer or when a woman might be, or is, pregnant or breastfeeding. Endometriosis, fibroids, gall bladder disease, undiagnosed vaginal bleeding and otosclerosis (an ear disorder) are other conditions where HRT may be inadvisable.

For many if not most other conditions specialist opinion suggests that HRT can be safely prescribed though each case should be individually considered. For example, most specialists now agree that even those who have high blood pressure can be given HRT once their blood pressure has been successfully treated and controlled. If your doctor won't prescribe HRT for you, do find out what the reasons are for this rather than wanting to change to another doctor on the spot! There may be a reason to do with your medical history which you haven't spotted and which he can point out to you.

WHAT IF I WANT TO COME OFF HRT?

If you develop unpleasant symptoms while taking HRT, this may be because you need to try another product. You can always ask your doctor to refer you to a specialist who will discuss other forms of HRT which may be better for you. He or she may propose altering the dosage from that which is normally recommended.

One leading consultant gynaecologist Malcolm Whitehead also suggests the following if you are having side-effects with HRT:

- If you get dyspepsia – indigestion– or other digestive upsets, try taking the tablets with food.
- If you have bad flushes during the day and bad sweats at night, maybe you could be given a divided daily dose of oestrogen to cover day and night. If the night sweats are worse you could take the tablets in the evening. If the daytime is worse you could take them in the morning.

Have some faith in what feels right for you. Your gut instinct may well be a good one. You know how your body feels better than anyone else. Balance all the information you have – it's important to get an all-round view, especially with the unrealistic expectations of perennial youth that may be floating around. Most women who take it thinking it will make them look young and glamorous stop taking it because it doesn't meet their dreams.

There can be side-effects and it is unrealistic to suggest otherwise. On the other hand there can be such huge benefits it would be a shame to let the potential side-effects sway someone in desperate need of help.

If you have been taking HRT and have decided to stop, it's important you talk to your doctor about this first. If a side-effect such as tender breasts is bothering you, for instance, your doctor should be able to reassure you that this often disappears after a few months as your body adjusts. According to one recent survey 80 per cent of women who had stopped taking HRT did so without informing their doctor. There may be alternatives to them stopping – a different prescription, for example. There may be useful information about their health that their doctor could give them. They may not have been taking it long enough for it to have an effect. To receive the full health benefits of HRT you may need to take it for at least two years. After ten years, the risks increase, particularly of breast cancer, but if you stop HRT after just a couple of years you are at much the same risk of heart disease and osteoporosis as if you had never taken it. If hot flushes are your problem, again you will probably need to take HRT for at least two years. If it's given for less time women have found the flushes do come back.

Whatever the case, if you go to your doctor to get put on long-term medication it makes sense to return to him or her if you want to stop taking it. If the prescription is right for the patient, doctors say they know of no other treatment which can make women feel so much better in so short a time. A month may be all it takes. So if you had hoped HRT was for you it's a shame if you don't give it a proper chance to help you out.

If you do decide you want to stop taking HRT, most doctors recommend this being a gradual process over about two months. Malcolm Whitehead, who's a big advocate of HRT, suggests taking a tablet every other day for three weeks, then one every fourth day – and that's only oestrogen tablets. Some doctors say you don't need to take progestogen while you are stopping but others say you do, so ask your doctor's advice. We think it better if you do.

Malcolm adds that many of those patients who decide

to stop taking HRT then come back again because their vagina feels dry. Maybe their flushes and sweats are not so bad but they find they have far less energy than they had when they were on the medication and that they can't concentrate as well. He says that for each woman who wants to stop, nine will want to start again.

To help you make your decision – or to help you learn more about the treatment you're receiving – here is a recap list of the possible benefits and risks of Hormone Replacement Therapy.

Benefits

- HRT appears to halt osteoporosis – the early thinning of the bones. It may prevent fractures of the bones in years to come. This benefit may be speculative for some as most women don't know if they will suffer from this condition. Also the protection stops when the treatment stops.

- It prevents heart disease – regarded by many doctors as the biggest health benefit. It's thought this is because it raises the concentration of the heart-protective HDL chemical in the bloodstream.

- It may prevent strokes. A team at Kings College Hospital found that it helps to keep the vital arteries supplying blood to the brain relaxed which means that circulation flows freely. Without this, the muscle walls would tense up more and more as the post-menopausal years go by. (You are roughly half as likely to die from a stroke or a heart attack if you take HRT.)

- It appears to help women suffering from various illnesses including rheumatoid arthritis, lupus and joint pains. Researchers are looking at why many women seem to get better when they take HRT and at the relationship between oestrogen and the immune system. It can be a huge relief when it no longer takes time to get the fingers and hands working in the mornings.

- It prevents hot flushes and night sweats.
- According to researchers in America it can help prevent Alzheimer's disease.
- If you suffer from migraines these should stop.
- It helps urinary problems such as cystitis and incontinence.
- It encourages the formation of collagen, keeping the skin elastic and young looking. It's not known if it actually prevents wrinkles.
- It keeps the vagina moist, making intercourse more comfortable.
- Especially if prescribed with a small amount of testosterone, the male hormone, it may bring back lost libido and so increase your sex drive.
- Self-confidence and a sense of well being can also increase.
- Some women say it gives them more energy.
- It helps you sleep better.
- It may help your battle against middle-age spread, as it stops fat building up around the stomach.
- You will get regular health checks – including mammograms and breast checks – so any problems will be caught quickly.

It can be less easy to take in fully the extent of the benefits because they can be benefits you might feel a long time into the future.

Risks

- There is thought to be a slightly increased risk of breast cancer, based largely, and perhaps falsely, on research on the contraceptive pill – another time when women are taking female hormones. Studies suggest that the increased risk is not a cause for concern until

HRT has been taken for more than ten years. However the increased risk is likely to encourage check-ups and could be better overall for the women taking HRT.

- Studies have suggested an increased risk of kidney complaints and liver complaints.
- You will usually continue to have a monthly bleed if you are taking the HRT which includes oestrogen and progestogen. This will be regular and will last around five days. This does put many women off. In fact because of this two out of three stop taking HRT within three years even if they feel good about its other effects and about themselves. The introduction of Livial – the brand which doesn't involve a monthly bleed – might make a big difference.
- You might continue to get symptoms like those of Pre-Menstrual Syndrome and tension before you bleed.
- There's a chance your breasts may swell up and become tender or you might find you're feeling sensitive around the nipples.
- Your ankles, too, may swell because of fluid retention and you may put on weight – though these symptoms are common at this time, even for women not taking HRT.
- You may suffer from mood swings and feel irritable.
- You may feel hungry at first.
- You may feel lethargic.
- You may feel bloated.
- Your blood pressure may rise.
- You may feel cramp in your calves.
- There might be a slightly increased risk of gall stones among younger women.

This might seem like a frightening list but, for most, these symptoms will only last a very short time. If they do not go away you can change to another HRT method which is more suitable for you. Of course not everyone gets all of these symptoms – many, if not most, women are aware of no negative effects of taking HRT at all and have been taking it for year after year very happily.

In our view, much of the research so far is inconclusive and does not, yet, take full account of the women not on HRT, who also get similar symptoms.

Lisa

One woman who felt the side-effects weren't worth it is Lisa. She's forty-five and a business woman and first went on HRT a year ago.

> I went on holiday with my boyfriend and nor-mally when we go away after a few days we really feel the benefits of lying on the beach. This time it was awful. I was bad-tempered the whole time, I had terrible pains in my legs which I put down to stress as I'd been very stressed when we left England.
>
> When I came back things were just as bad. I'd be crying in the office or losing my temper for no reason. I felt awful afterwards, losing control like that, upsetting the harmony of the office. They'd be sitting there thinking, 'What mood is she in today?' I'd slam the phone down on someone and then they'd know.
>
> Up to that point I'd just thought, 'I need a holiday,' but since the holiday nothing had changed. One morning at work I had to leave the office and walk around outside after losing my temper over nothing. It was like the worst PMT I have ever had. I stood in a shop looking at people and just thought I was going mad. I went back to the office and signed myself out for the rest of the day.
>
> My period didn't come and at that point I

realised I had a problem. I started to read up on the change of life.

Lisa told her doctor her symptoms, which by this stage also included bad headaches. She was prescribed HRT.

The doctor said I would notice an effect quite quickly and I did. For the first few months there was a distinct improvement. I looked a lot better and I started to lose weight. My interest in sex had returned and I was feeling better about myself and my body.

Then after three months I went back to square one. I was down, feeling sluggish, couldn't sleep and I was eating a lot. I was fighting with my boyfriend all the time, not sleeping and going to work feeling tired.

Lisa went back for a different dosage.

I wasn't expecting miracles – I don't think you can from pills – but I was prepared to give it another go. I felt bloated and was still eating too much – sweet things all the time. Some days I felt better but not enough for me to persevere with it. I read somewhere that not everyone is suited to HRT and maybe that's me. Maybe I should concentrate on better diet and more exercise and a more healthy lifestyle.

My boyfriend kept nagging me to stop. Every time we had a row it would be, 'Those damn pills.'

I'm usually quite a decisive person but in the past twelve months I've been unable to make a single decision, or that's how it feels. Until now that is. Now I've made the decision to come off HRT and try to look after myself better.

As I mentioned earlier, there's been press coverage about the risk of addiction to HRT – reports that oestrogen is as addictive as heroin or cocaine and that women find they have withdrawal symptoms unless their dosage is increased. It's been suggested that the powerful psychological effect of HRT could encourage dependency. But we believe it's more likely that women feel so much better when they're taking HRT that they don't want to stop and, frankly, we can't see much wrong with that.

And we'd like to repeat that while you are taking HRT you will have to be under the supervision of your doctor. Even if everything is going swimmingly and you feel you have no problems at all, you need to see your doctor every six months. He or she might wish to do a mammogram, test your blood pressure and maybe examine you internally. You will certainly be carefully monitored and looked after.

Of course the issue of breast cancer is the biggest one on our list of risks. Breast cancer is a huge issue for women, for reasons of femininity as well as health. The breast is where cancer most commonly strikes a woman and there are about 25,000 new cases every year – one in fourteen women will suffer from the disease. For those fifty-five and over the death rate from breast cancer rises from two per thousand to three per thousand among HRT users and that is a significant increase.

Malcolm Whitehead says that if a patient's mother developed breast cancer before her menopause, that may double the patient's risk of developing breast cancer. She is certainly at a greater risk than if her mother developed the disease after the menopause, so that's something to bear in mind.

It's ironic that progestogen is taken with oestrogen to stop cancer of the womb because it's thought to be progestogen which might increase the risk of breast cancer, a much more common disease.

Look after your breasts. Get to know them and check them as described in the next chapter and ask to be sent for a mammogram at least every three years. If you notice anything different or worrying about your breasts go to your GP and if you are on HRT remind him or her of that when you discuss what you've noticed.

And don't be too alarmed. You probably need to have been taking HRT for ten years before the breast cancer risk is real. Also worth bearing in mind is that for every case of cancer, six deaths are saved from bone fractures, strokes and heart disease – the advantages of HRT heavily outweigh the disadvantages.

As with everything else in life, we have to balance the risks we take against what we might gain. With HRT, the benefits in quality of life have been enormous. Sometimes the relief felt has been instantaneous. And some women have taken HRT for twenty years or more with no known ill-effects.

Of course it's not a miracle cure, the answer to all our problems. Once Valium and other tranquillisers were handed out all too easily to conceal psychological problems and there have been suggestions HRT might be doing the same. It is easier, after all, to take extra hormones than to dig deeper at causes of depression. It could also be argued that if you lost your self-esteem and self-confidence at the time of the menopause, maybe it was shaky in the first place. HRT will only help if your depression has a hormonal basis. Otherwise counselling and therapy might be more helpful and effective solutions.

Similarly with sexual problems. If dryness is a major problem, HRT will be a plus. But sexual problems are often a mirror of other problems in a relationship. If you and your partner are not communicating well, HRT won't suddenly make you want to have lots of sex with him. And please don't forget, HRT is not a contraceptive and you should keep using a form of contraception until one year after your last period if you're over fifty, two years if you're under fifty unless your doctor tells you otherwise.

Whatever you do, don't suffer in silence. HRT can be individually tailored for the individual woman. The ratio of oestrogen to progestogen can be changed. You can try the recommended alternative methods of receiving the hormones. You can try Livial and avoid the monthly bleeds. Tell your doctor what your symptoms are and ask not only for his advice but also for what you want.

Otherwise you can turn to a local Well Woman Clinic or menopause clinic for advice. These are usually available under the NHS. Or you could go to the Margaret Pyke Centre in Soho (for address see page 95) – which is also an NHS clinic and offers a menopause service. The centre is especially aware of the needs of the older women. As their ovaries begin to work less well (often 5–10 years before their actual last period) and they may come to need oestrogens, they also need to have absolute confidence that they won't have an unexpected and unwanted pregnancy. So the MPC provides a special and most comprehensive service for women approaching the menopause. They call these clinic sessions the '40'-plus clinics' and they are staffed entirely by women.

Beyond the menopause, although women need oestrogen to help their hearts and bones and general well-being, they don't particularly like continuing to have periods. So MPC is studying ways to get all the benefits without getting any bleeding at all, using a special device that protects and prevents bleeding from the womb while still allowing oestrogen to be given by any chosen route. This device should be widely available in 1994, but attendance at the MPC may, in appropriate cases, allow it to be used sooner. There is an Advice Sister service too, to answer urgent telephone enquiries or supply walk-in advice about family planning and HRT. All this is available free of charge on the NHS, as we have said, and without the need for an initial letter from a doctor – you just get in touch.

Alternatively, you could contact the Amarant Centre which was established in central London in 1987 at the Churchill Clinic because of the demand of women who wanted expert and sympathetic help during their menopause and couldn't find it elsewhere. Thousands of women have since walked through their doors from all over the country. They also have advice lines to ring (see the list at the end of this book). It's not part of the NHS although it is staffed by specialists trained at Kings College Hospital. You do have to pay for its services but you might be covered by private medical insurance.

You can either ask your GP to refer you to the Centre or you can go straight there yourself and they will contact your GP for permission to treat you. To make a claim on your medical insurance you must have been referred there by your GP.

Once you get there you will have a consultation which will take about an hour. You'll be seen by a nursing sister and a specialist doctor and you'll talk about your health, your symptoms and your medical history. You'll have a physical examination and a discussion about the risks and benefits of HRT and other treatments. There will be plenty of time for you to ask questions and say how you feel.

You may have to have further tests – either through your GP or at the Amarant Centre itself. Otherwise, if it's appropriate, you may be prescribed HRT immediately. You then go back for your second appointment in three months and a third in six months. If necessary your treatment will be adjusted. After this you go back every six months or you go for a check-up to your GP, whichever you prefer.

Sometimes they recommend hormone tests, especially if you have symptoms such as hot flushes, night sweats and vaginal dryness and yet you are not responding to HRT, or if there is a question mark over whether hormone deficiency is the cause of your problems. They may also recommend hormone tests in women whose menopause seems to be starting early to check whether your symptoms are due to hormone deficiency.

At the Centre they also have facilities to carry out bone density scans, endometrial biopsies which check the lining of the womb for abnormalities, mammograms, pelvic ultrasound to check on abnormal swellings or enlargements of ovaries or womb, a full blood count to check for anaemia, tests for the function of the liver and thyroid, a lipid profile to check cholesterol and a thrombotic-risk profile.

So, if you like the idea of HRT, why not try it and see. It's a decision many women are delighted they made.

Chapter Three
SELF-HELP TREATMENT

The menopause, as we've said, is a natural stage in a woman's life. It's not a disease or an illness. It's not something bad which makes female bodies fall apart and minds fall to pieces. It's an inevitable part of women's lives, a very personal and a very complicated part.

Because of this it's vital that you allow time to yourself, that you put yourself first and decide what you want and need to help you cope well and look forward to the future.

We feel clear that Hormone Replacement Therapy can be a huge boost for women who are finding their menopause difficult to cope with and for those who want to protect their longer-term health. But we also feel it would be a shame if HRT was presented as the only option. After all, every woman's menopause is different; and every woman's attitude to health and life is different too. Certainly the complete medicalisation of all our lives would be a narrow-minded way to look at how we can improve our lot and learn to be healthier and happier.

RECOGNISE YOUR NEEDS

One of the best medicines of all is free if you go to the right places, and you don't even need a prescription. We're talking about sympathy and understanding – always a great tonic. It's very common for women to suffer in silence, to see themselves as there for their husband and children, giving emotional and physical support whenever it's needed. It may well be that it's you who needs that support now and the best way to receive it is to ask for it. Telling the people around you how you feel is a vital way to help them understand you and your emotions. Even if you think a relationship is crumbling, even if you're feeling so depressed you don't believe anyone could help or understand, the worst thing you can do is keep it to yourself.

And if you do decide to express your feelings, think hard about who it would be best to confide in. Talk to those who will be sympathetic rather than those who may want to run your life for you and present you with all the answers. Talk to someone who will be listening to you rather than someone waiting for you to pause for breath so they can have their say. Choose someone who won't judge you and won't put you down, someone who preferably won't be distracted by children running round them asking for biscuits or who won't have to dash out to catch the shops before you've finished.

Talk to someone who'll listen with both ears. If your husband's muttering to you in response while still watching the television or reading the newspaper, this won't help you feel your problems and needs are important. Tell him what you want – ten undistracted minutes of his time, perhaps, for him to listen to what you have to say.

An alternative to expressing your feelings is to take the Trojan, stiff-upper-lip path. This would entail telling yourself that the symptoms you're suffering are only to be expected. No one else is complaining so why should you? And in any case they'll disappear sooner or later after your body is used to the changes so there's no point making a fuss. If you're feeling like this you'll probably be especially scathing of your psychological symptoms. A headache's a headache, there's no getting away from that, but if you can't remember anything you're meant to be doing and your concentration's gone completely you may find it harder to be kind to yourself.

If there are other things in your life causing you stress, try writing them all down. That act by itself may help you to deal with them, rather than allowing them to overwhelm you.

When you're not feeling great – especially if you're tired, run down and depressed – it's easy to fail to spend this sort of time on yourself. It's also easy not to spend the time to buy and cook and eat nourishing food, wear the clothes you feel good in, or wash your hair as often as you'd like. All of this will make you feel less energised and even more run down. Your symptoms will get worse and your resistance to them will be less.

There are one or two common sense ideas which can help to make life more pleasant – wearing several layers of light clothing rather than one big jumper so you can remove some of your layers during a hot flush and put them back on afterwards, and concentrating on cotton garments without high necks, are straightforward suggestions but ones which might not occur to you if you're feeling too run down to give yourself the attention you deserve and need.

FOOD AND DRINK

It is suggested that as we get older we need more balanced meals, for example, more fibre for a healthy bowel and vitamin-rich foods. We should get enough vitamins if we eat a wide variety of foods and don't get into a 'rut' – the white bread and tea syndrome. Our bodies can cope less well with heavily fatty junk food since after the menopause women need fewer calories and less protein too – they're no longer menstruating and their muscles are not so active.

It is claimed that too much animal protein is a bad idea as this leads to calcium being excreted in the urine. For this reason, it is said, meat-eaters can be more likely to get osteoporosis than vegetarians, although we're not convinced about this.

To keep bones strong a diet high in calcium is recommended. It's found in milk, cheese and other dairy products, seafood, seeds and root vegetables. Low-fat dairy produce is healthier than the full-fat variety and there are plenty of different brands and products on the market these days.

According to the National Osteoporosis Society, a good calcium-rich diet should include at least three servings a day from milk group foods such as a glass of milk, a carton of yogurt or two ounces of cheese (Cheddar, Gouda and Edam are ideal). Nuts, tinned salmon and sardines (including all the bones), many dark green leafy vegetables, such as kale and broccoli, and dried fruits are other foods which are good for bones. If you can't tolerate dairy products, goat's milk and cheese are an alternative, but they are very fatty. Calcium enriched soya milk is another option. An extra advantage of dairy produce is that, along with sunflower seeds, it contains a lot of vitamin E which is useful in reducing hot flushes and alleviating vaginal dryness (also true of vitamins B and C). Vitamin C helps absorb the calcium found in fruit and vegetables.

To make depression less likely you could try eating foods containing high quantities of magnesium and calcium. These include fish, root vegetables, nuts and meat. Bananas are also alleged to have this effect because of the Tryptophan they contain. Magnesium is found in green vegetables and also in brown rice and wholewheat bread – far more so than in their white counterparts. Nuts, seeds and grains contain magnesium too. Always be careful not to overcook green vegetables or they will lose their nutritional value.

Roger Stanway, who wrote *Diet for Common Ailments* (published by Sidgwick and Jackson, 1989) which has a section on the menopause, suggests keeping away from animal fats as there is a rise in blood fats in the body after the menopause. He says raw fruit and vegetables, nuts and grains have a natural oestrogenic effect. He also advises a diet which includes foods rich in fatty acids such as seeds, nuts, wheatgerm, tomatoes, peppers and garlic and he's another advocate of vitamin C, found in great quantities in citrus fruits and juices and leafy green vegetables. Vitamin D-rich foods are important for absorbing calcium in the intestine and strengthening bones. They include egg yolks, liver, fortified milk, cereals and salt water fish.

Looking after the heart is important after the menopause when women no longer have their high levels of naturally produced oestrogen to protect them. And, for many women, the post-menopausal years are less active, which has a negative effect on the heart, and as we get older our heart becomes more vulnerable. However, HRT does lessen the risk of heart disease.

The British Heart Foundation advocates a diet which helps with weight loss and which reduces blood cholesterol levels. Its general rule is to cut down on fat, particularly animal fats, which will help with weight and cholesterol. Cream, full-cream milk, many cheeses, cakes, biscuits and fatty meat are sources of fat which can be reduced. On the other hand the Foundation recommends increasing the amount of oily fish and some cooking oils. It also suggests increasing the intake of fresh fruit and vegetables to five portions a day. Cutting down on salt is important, especially if your blood pressure is higher than average. Cutting down on sugar doesn't have a particular link to helping the heart, unless you eat too much which will give you a bigger chance of becoming obese, of developing diabetes and of aggravating arthritis.

The British Heart Foundation quotes the following weight chart produced by the Scottish Health Education Group, which should give you some idea of whether you need to lose weight.

Height	Average weight	Acceptable weight range	Obese
4ft 10in	7st 4lb	6st 8lb–8st 7lb	10st 3lb
4ft 11in	7st 6lb	6st 10lb–8st 10lb	10st 6lb
5ft	7st 9lb	6st 12lb–8st 13lb	10st 10lb
5ft 1in	7st 12lb	7st 1lb–9st 2lb	11st
5ft 2in	8st 1lb	7st 4lb–9st 5lb	11st 3lb
5ft 3in	8st 4lb	7st 7lb–9st 8lb	11st 7lb
5ft 4in	8st 8lb	7st 10lb–9st 12lb	11st 12lb
5ft 5in	8st 11lb	7st 13lb–10st 2lb	12st 2lb
5ft 6in	9st 2lb	8st 2lb–10st 6lb	12st 7lb
5ft 7in	9st 6lb	8st 6lb–10st 10lb	12st 12lb
5ft 8in	9st 10lb	8st 10lb–11st	13st 3lb
5ft 9in	10st	9st–11st 4lb	13st 8lb
5ft 10in	10st 4lb	9st 4lb–11st 9lb	14st
5ft 11in	10st 8lb	9st 8lb–12st	14st 6lb
6ft	10st 12lb	9st 12lb–12st 5lb	14st 12lb

If you have any worries about dieting and whether it's right for you, ask your GP for advice. It's important that even when you are on a diet you are consuming enough calcium and see that vitamins are included.

A moderate amount of alcoholic drink may give some

protection against heart attacks. However, you shouldn't increase your intake on that account. If you never or rarely drink you shouldn't increase your drinking. Women should stick to a maximum of two drinks a day – that's the equivalent of a pint of beer, a double measure of spirits or two glasses of wine.

If you want to prevent osteoporosis don't drink too much caffeine as this increases calcium loss. Coffee is the worst culprit but tea and cocoa also have to be watched, especially in large quantities. Alcohol and fizzy drinks – even fizzy water – are also said to add to the problem. There's an interesting claim that in America one of the causes of osteoporosis is fizzy drinks which contain phosphorous as phosphorous decreases the amount of calcium in the body.

Alcohol and coffee are also bad news if you are suffering from hot flushes so they are best avoided at these times. Alcohol may also stop the liver processing vitamin D if you drink to excess.

Finally, a postscript. If you overdo the food and drink and want to take antacids, take those based on magnesium rather than on aluminium or sodium if you are of menopausal age. Other drugs, mainly the prescribed steroids, can have a negative effect on the bones as well.

SUPPLEMENTS

A favourite for those who don't want to take hormones is boron. This has some very staunch supporters – although we are not among them! – and advocates claim it helps women through the menopause. It's a mineral available in health shops, and is found in its natural form in salads, green vegetables and fruit.

There is still much confusion about the value of this supplement but what does make sense is that good nutrition can improve oestrogen levels even after the menopause, which is an exciting thought.

If you have a history of osteoporosis in your family, sometimes supplements are recommended. Calcium supplements with added vitamins A and D plus magnesium are suggested to slow down possible osteoporosis development. Even from as young as your mid-twenties there's an argument that supplements will keep your bones strong and be a good preparation for your later years. However taking calcium in supplement form after the menopause might not help because oestrogen is needed for calcium to be absorbed and, of course, after the menopause the oestrogen required isn't around. Some experts say calcium supplements are only useful and necessary if, for some reason, your diet tends to be inadequate as far as calcium is concerned. Other medical experts have yet another view – they question whether eating calcium-rich foods and taking supplements have any positive effect on post-menopausal bones and suggest instead that exercise is the most helpful way of strengthening our skeletons (see page 76-7).

Vitamin D is especially important to ensure good calcium uptake. Sunshine is a vital element in providing vitamin D and in the United Kingdom, where sunshine is often lacking, a supplement of this vitamin may occasionally be advised for those who cannot go out easily, for example. The disabled and the elderly who don't go out much and who also may not get as much exercise are particularly at risk from a lack of vitamin D.

However too much vitamin D is bad for the bones, according to the National Osteoporosis Society, who warn that it's important not to go over the recommended amount, which is four hundred international units a day. More than this can be toxic – a doubling of the recommended limit can cause kidney stones. The Society says the vitamin does help with the absorption of calcium in the intestine and it does strengthen bones but most people get enough from being outside and from vitamin D-rich foods.

Then we also need magnesium in order to metabolise the calcium, and a shortage of magnesium is very common. Some of the symptoms of magnesium deficiency, according to the British Society for Nutritional Medicine, are poor memory, inability to sleep, fatigue, apathy and palpitations. Again, the medical evidence for this is lacking – unless the sufferer is starting, or on, a crank diet!

Some women swear by multi-vitamin and mineral tablets which they say have removed their symptoms. Some, such as Confiance are specially formulated to help women through the menopause. Other women advocate Ginseng and Royal Jelly.

Some menopausal women still suffer from Pre-Menstrual Syndrome and Pre-Menstrual Tension. This means your ovaries are still secreting hormones – although not in big enough quantities to give you periods – so you experience tension, depression, irritability, tears, rages, tender breasts, headaches or insomnia. If this is the case, try Evening Primrose Oil and vitamin B6, especially if these worked for you while you were menstruating. Vitamin B complex tablets generally help your nervous system to function well.

Vitamins C and E and Evening Primrose Oil are all worth a try. In fact, E is said to promote the production of oestrogen naturally. Vitamin C is essential in the formation of collagen which is needed for skin elasticity and bones.

Another useful supplement is that of fluoride in drinking water, which is good for bones as well as teeth.

Generally we feel happier with the thought of a healthy, varied, wholesome diet than we do with popping lots of different vitamin pills and mineral supplements.

However at this stage in your life, added vitamins and minerals may give you a much needed boost. Be careful not to overdo it, though. By increasing your intake you won't feel better; in fact you may make yourself feel worse. Check the sides of packets for recommended dosage and, if in doubt, buy from a pharmacy and seek the pharmacist's professional advice.

Hazel

Hazel found some relief in taking B vitamins for her menopausal symptoms which were extreme.

> It felt as if my brain wasn't working properly, as if I was having some sort of breakdown. It was like I had a double personality. I couldn't bear to go out on my own. It got to the point where I couldn't stand at my sink and wash up. I'd stand there with a cloth in my hand and a plate in the water and think, 'What am I supposed to do with this?' I didn't know how to wash up!
>
> My mind would throw me false information. It was like living in a waking nightmare. I'd be watching a nature programme on the television about Africa and giraffes and then I'd think, 'Why are they there? Why's that lion there? Why are those people there? Why have they made this programme?' I was asking questions there were no answers to.
>
> I went to my doctor who gave me an extra-long appointment and he told me he felt my problem was hormone imbalance. I couldn't believe it – I thought he was going to lock me up in a straitjacket!
>
> He said he'd put me on some B6 which would help the logical side of my brain to work properly

as well as some other B vitamins. This helped enormously.

The problem with B6 is that it builds up toxins in the body and so I only stayed on it for six or eight months, but long enough to feel like a human being again.

Hazel moved on to herbal remedies with vitamins and minerals and now runs the organisation Mid-Life Matters (see page 95 for address) which supplies specially formulated packages of herbs, vitamins and minerals to menopausal women. She doesn't believe in HRT, which she says is synthetic and which she feels puts off what's natural and inevitable. 'I don't see why we should have a false bleed and delay nature. Why not,' she asks, 'find something to help you get through what nature intended you to?' She did, although sometimes she still gets symptoms.

Still very occasionally when I'm out I start to panic. I dive out of shops because I can't bear to be there. And I'm not alone. You can tell by the number of full and abandoned supermarket trolleys.

Again, though we aren't convinced that Hazel has all the answers or that her theories are fully supportable, she's found ways to cope with her problems – and, if you can do this safely, we wouldn't quarrel with that.

EXERCISE

OK, OK, don't groan. We're aware the worst possible thing to suggest to someone who doesn't exercise is lots of exercise so we're not going to do that.

But exercising *is* good for you, not just for your all-round health, but for your bones, your heart, your moods, and your energy levels – a lot of important areas for menopausal women. And you may find that regular exercise replaces other life rhythms which you no longer have during and after the menopause.

Our theory is that a bit of exercise every day is better than an all-out sweaty session which leaves you feeling totally exhausted. If you're not doing any exercise at the moment then take it gently. Go for a short swim or a bit of a brisk walk. You'll be amazed how good this keeps you feeling about yourself and how much it adds to your energy. As well as this, it's good for your bones – and that's especially true of stretching exercises, for when muscles stretch and contract this applies pressure to the bones and they become stronger.

Exercise that bears your weight is good for you too, so something as straightforward as walking is ideal. Or you could try tennis, badminton, gentle jogging or dancing to keep your bones strong. Remember bones are made up of living tissue and they deteriorate if they're not used, just as muscles sag through lack of use. This is especially worth keeping in mind for those of us with a basically sedentary lifestyle. A walk has another benefit too – a lack of daylight is not good for us and, even when it's cloudy, rays of light come from the sun that trigger in us the formation of vitamin D which is so vital for the absorption of calcium.

Studies funded by the group Research into Ageing and the Oxford Regional Health Authority, and carried out at Ealing and Hammersmith Hospitals, suggest that exercise can preserve and increase the amount of bone in the skeleton. The research shows that a bone reacts to the forces put on it by maintaining enough bone mineral to withstand those forces. However many activities which put a stress on bones are no longer with us – such as wringing out huge piles of washing and carrying heavy loads. The findings suggest that if you spend a minute or two a week struggling with an activity which your bones find difficult it helps retain their density and strength. 'For most people carrying something which they find heavy, preferably up a few steps and as briskly as possible, should do the trick,' says Michael Beverly, the consultant surgeon involved. His trials showed that when these exercises which stressed the bones were stopped, the gains were lost. Another study in America showed that vigorously exercising for an hour a day increased bone calcium by up to a third in menopausal women.

For exercise to help the heart it has to be vigorous enough to make you slightly breathless. It also has to be carried out regularly – around twenty to thirty minutes' worth three times a week. Work up gradually to this and don't do more than you can manage. If you're at all worried about whether you should be exercising, ask your doctor what he or she thinks.

Generally, when you're thinking about exercise, choose a routine which you think will be suitable for you. Don't decide on an incredibly strenuous daily keep-fit routine if you know in your heart you won't keep it up and will lose the enthusiasm and good will you started with.

Something ideal might be stretching exercises or swimming which will improve your breathing and your circulation. You don't have to 'feel the burn', we're not talking from the 'no pain no gain' school of fitness. Wherever you are, whether in the swimming pool or in the aerobics class, don't be put off if others seem to be better than you. Exercise isn't about competing but about what each of us can do for ourselves.

Ideally, you will have begun exercising before the menopause. Again this doesn't have to mean a fearsome aerobics class filled with twenty-year-olds in Lycra leotards and leggings. If you prefer, it doesn't even have to mean leaving the house any more than you would normally. It can mean walking up stairs instead of taking lifts or escalators, dancing at home with children or grandchildren or by yourself, walking instead of taking the car on short journeys. If you feel you can do more still, think about going on longer walks, maybe joining a stretch exercise or other keep-fit class, playing tennis, swimming or badminton. Try to make it part of a well-rounded way of life which gives you energy and vitality rather than something you have to force yourself to do.

Exercising a few times a week will cut down on your tension levels and on any feelings you may have of being 'past it'. There's also that great 'after glow' when you've finished, when you're slightly breathless and realise what you've achieved.

Yoga is a great form of exercise, too, and has many benefits, especially the wonderful feeling of calm it can induce.

PROTECT YOUR BACK AND AVOID ACCIDENTS

A firm bed is very good for your back – especially if osteoporosis is present. If you don't have one and can't afford to buy a new mattress try putting a sheet of stiff plywood underneath your present mattress. Cheap but quite effective.

Be careful when lifting heavy objects, bending at the knees so you are using the strength in your legs without straining your back. Many small fractures of the spine are the result of not doing this.

Try to move position as often as you can. Sitting for very long periods can put a strain on the back.

Make sure the edges of carpets and rugs can't be tripped over. They can be secured to the floor to prevent accidents. Tidiness is a good safety measure. If children's toys are lying around they should be put in a corner out of harm's way and the same goes for garden equipment which can be hidden in grass. Rooms should be organised so electrical and telephone wires aren't draped across pathways.

Always use a small step-ladder when trying to reach a high cupboard or shelf – don't balance on a stool, chair or anything else not meant for the purpose. So many accidents are caused this way.

Slippery surfaces are another hazard. So if liquids are spilt on the floor they should be wiped up straight away. Keep snow and ice cleared as much as possible and don't over-polish floors. Non-slip stickers in baths are a good idea. So are handles fixed to the sides to help you get in and out without mishap.

STOP SMOKING

Smoking is bad news for many, many reasons, but here we're talking about one which gets less publicity: if you smoke your menopause comes, on average, two years earlier. This means your body will have two extra years without the benefits which its natural hormones should provide.

Cigarettes also can cause outbreaks of sweating and hot flushes – another good reason for quitting. If you can't do it by yourself there are some very good books available to help you do this, as well as nicotine substitutes available from chemists. If you still can't manage to give up, you may find acupuncture can help relieve your withdrawal symptoms so it may be worth giving that a try (see page 86).

We've been writing about the possibly increased risk of breast cancer and of uterine cancer which might come from the prolonged use of HRT. Yet nothing does more to prevent cancer than giving up smoking, so we feel it's important to get this into context.

We've also talked of heart disease and the potential benefits of HRT. Yet smoking positively causes heart disease and, if we're worried about our future health, stopping smoking is an excellent step towards looking after our bodies and ourselves.

RELAXATION

We're pretty sure that the more women worry about the effects of the menopause and what the symptoms might have in store for them next, the worse things are going to be.

Relaxation is one of the keys to coping with a troublesome menopause. So if you feel a flush coming on, relax and try to let yourself 'go with it' rather than fight it. It's better to allow yourself to sweat for a few minutes than to tense up or panic. Placing a fan on your desk if you work in an office might help you to do this comfortably. If you feel very uncomfortable, try placing the insides of your wrists and arms on a cold surface or under a cold tap.

A couple of years ago we watched a television interview with the Body Shop's Anita Roddick and remember her saying that sun, smoke and stress did more harm to the skin than anything else. So relaxation has more benefits than the simple and admirable aim of peace of mind.

Relaxation classes are ideal. Your local education authority might run some. Otherwise, even if life feels crazily busy, just giving yourself a quarter of an hour of peace and quiet and time for your own thoughts can be rejuvenating and relaxing. Few things in life are so urgent they can't wait a quarter of an hour.

Try simple breathing exercises: breathing in slowly through your nose, out through your mouth. Maybe you could do this while visualising a favourite peaceful place. Another idea is to tense and release all parts of your body one after the other, from the tips of your fingers to the tips of your toes.

Massage can be very relaxing for the muscles and the mind. As well as this it improves circulation and releases fluid from the tissues. This ensures a better flow of blood to the brain and so an improved supply of nutrients to the brain which is good for any mental imbalance.

Another great way of relaxing is making love – if you feel relaxed with your partner, that is. Give yourselves time. Plan this so there won't be interruptions and other matters on your minds. If your vagina is dry you may find you need more foreplay than before to stimulate you. KY jelly applied to the vulva and the vagina may be a help if you still feel too dry for comfortable sex. Frequent intercourse should keep the walls of the vagina stronger.

If you have problems with periods or are suffering a great deal of fatigue, or you have resentments towards your partner, you may feel you don't want to have sex. If that's OK for both of you that's fine. Otherwise it is always a good idea to talk about what's happening in the physical side of your relationship rather than just allow things to slide.

As an added bonus, any form of warm physical contact, from sex to a hug to a massage, is a great aid to a good night's sleep.

A long soak in the bath can be a good, peaceful way to relax, especially if the phone's off the hook and you're not expecting any visitors. If you're having problems with vaginal dryness we'd advise you not to use any perfumed soaps or bubble baths as this might aggravate your condition.

Another great way to relax is to have fun. If you can't remember the last time you did that, it's worth reorganising some of your priorities. A good giggle at a television programme might be all you need to lighten your load and help put troubles into perspective.

POSITIVE THINKING

At this time in your life positive thinking will be a big plus. After all, other places in the world don't value youthful beauty more than the maturity and experience of old age, and why should we? It's no surprise that in countries where middle-aged women have less standing there are more menopausal problems.

Low self-esteem is at the root of so many emotional problems, and raising it isn't easy by yourself, but trying to listen to positive messages you receive rather than critical ones is a start. There are very good books available which can help us take charge of our lives and stop us blaming others for our misfortunes. Most book shops have a section which stocks self-help type books.

Achievements always make us feel good and if you are unstimulated in your life and don't have enough to fill your day and utilise your talents, that's a recipe for feeling down and unmotivated. Depression isn't always hormonal, far from it, and if you're feeling low a counsellor or psychotherapist might help you see what you can do to change your life.

You may have disappointments but try to think also about the achievements you've accomplished. In most events in life there is good as well as bad. Maybe this time could be like a plateau in your life to give you the space and perspective to look back and look forward. Maybe there are elements to your life now you've never had before – more financial security perhaps, more time for yourself, no contraceptive worries, no period pains. Whatever. Positive thinking isn't always easy but it's the most constructive, optimistic way to live our lives, so give it a try. If you can't, maybe you might benefit from some extra support and guidance to help you on your way in life.

BREAST CARE

The age group when women take HRT is the age group when women tend to get breast cancer – that is from the late forties to around sixty. So it's important all women are aware of any changes in their body or in their breasts which are unusual for them. Check them and get them checked.

It's no longer specifically recommended that women check their breasts at particular intervals, although if you do give yourself regular breast checks, that's fine. The mood now is for women to become more familiar with their bodies, something they haven't always been encouraged to do. The influence of feminism changed this but many still don't touch and look and stand naked in front of their mirrors. If a woman is aware of her body – how she feels without touching, whether her breasts ache, how they feel to the touch and how they look – she's much more likely to notice changes. When you soap down under the shower or in the bath or when you're dressing, see if you notice any slight differences. If you do, mention them to your doctor.

Remember if you're still having your periods your breasts will feel different at the various times of your monthly cycle. Before your period starts your milk-producing tissue becomes activated and this means breasts can feel tender and lumpy. This is especially true of the areas near the armpits.

After your menopause the breasts will tend to feel softer and they won't feel lumpy as the milk-producing process isn't happening any more. They will be less firm than before. If you've had a hysterectomy it's likely your breasts will continue to have the same monthly changes as before, until the time your periods would have stopped naturally.

Be aware if your nipples are inverted when they usually aren't, if you have lumps, or puckering of the skin surface, or a spot that won't go away. It's always worth getting a doctor to look at it.

The National Health Service Breast Screening Programme suggests you look out for the following changes:

- Appearance. Look for any change in the outline or shape of the breast, especially those caused by arm movements or by lifting the breasts. Look for any puckering or dimpling of the skin.
- Feelings. Check whether you are aware of any discomfort or pain which is different from normal, especially if it is new and persistent.
- Lumps. See if there are any lumps, thickening or bumpy areas in one breast or armpit which seem to be different from the same part of the other breast and armpit. This is very important if it is a new development.
- Nipple change. Look for nipple discharge that's new for you and not milky. Look out for bleeding or moist, reddish areas which don't heal easily. Also look out for any change in nipple position – it might be pulled in or pointing in a different direction. Also check for a rash on or around the nipple.

Remember, if you find a lump that doesn't necessarily

mean you have cancer. Nine out of ten lumps aren't cancerous. If you're under forty, breast cancer is rare.

If you do have a little lump, it's worth knowing about it. Don't let fear keep you away from your doctor. Let him or her decide whether it's significant or not. And, if it is cancer, it's far better that it's dealt with as early as possible.

Chapter Four
ALTERNATIVE THERAPIES

ACUPUNCTURE

This is a traditional Chinese medicine and increasing numbers of women report that it has given them relief from menopausal symptoms.

The theory behind it is that Chi – vital energy – flows in our bodies, concentrated in meridians or vertical paths. Emotional and physical factors can restrict this flow which affects our well-being and energy levels.

Acupuncture helps in maintaining general health and is also good for relieving specific symptoms. It treats one of the most common problems, hot flushes, using the triple heater meridian which, according to Chinese medical theory, regulates the flow of temperature between the three parts of the body – the upper, middle and lower parts. You can see how different this theory is from the Western approach.

Acupuncture can treat women suffering insomnia and restlessness and is used in conjunction with self-help advice – not drinking coffee and doing relaxation exercises are popular suggestions. The feelings of dizziness that often come with the menopause are put down to changes going on in the liver which can be treated with Chinese herbal medicine. Low libido and forgetfulness can, say practitioners, also be effectively dealt with. Acupuncturists suggest coming to them regularly before you approach the menopause. In fact a lot of women go for treatment for menstrual problems. The practitioners say if you have acupuncture on a regular basis beforehand, together with a good diet and exercise, your transition through will be smoother.

Acupuncture can be combined with Western medicines – even with HRT. If you are worried about the slight increase in cancer risk associated with HRT, oriental medicine links cancer risks with stagnation and acupuncture is said to keep the body flowing by stimulating all its systems.

Many people are put off by the thought of being pricked by needles, but this isn't like an injection. The needles are of hairlike thinness and sometimes aren't felt at all as they're inserted. Of course it's nothing like the sort of treatment we were brought up to expect from medical experts but we know many people who swear by it and some GPs are also trained acupuncture practitioners.

HERBALISM

Herbalist Anne McIntyre says her form of therapy has been very successful in treating women with menopausal symptoms. She starts off by taking a general case history of the patient to work out why they are suffering from the symptoms.

She looks for the reasons why these women in particular are feeling the symptoms when others go through their menopause without these sorts of problems. 'They could have a history of hormone imbalance. There could be a hereditary factor – their mother or grandmother may have had them. Very often women with menopausal problems have had problems in the past with their periods or have generally had a difficult or stressful time over the past few years. I think stress directly affects hormonal balance so I treat with herbs not only the hormonal balance but also the nervous system.'

Anne also looks at the woman's diet and her lifestyle. 'There might not be enough in her diet to support her nervous system or her hormonal system. When you're going through a period of change you need support from your diet. You need plenty of vitamin E and B and polyunsaturated fats which have essential fatty acids. You also need calcium and magnesium and I'd rather they got to grips with their diet than had supplements although I might suggest these for a short period of time.'

Anne, whose practice is in the Cotswolds, treats her clients with herbs and says she's very surprised if their symptoms don't get better without the need for HRT. Herbalists use camomile to help with tiredness and sensitivity and recommend sage and nettle teas for anyone going through the menopause as they're rich in substances said to correspond to female hormones. Anne might use skullcap and vervain for the nervous system and, specifically for menopausal depression and for feelings of vulnerability and insecurity, she might use St John's Wort. Wild oats, lemon balm and rosemary also support the nervous system. She might suggest sage and motherwort for hot flushes and thyme for nervous problems. Hot flushes can also be treated with chaste tree, yarrow, wormwood, lady's slipper or mistletoe. Chaste tree is one of the major hormone-balancing herbs that Anne uses, which is said to work on the pituitary gland and sexual hormones. Another, False Unicorn Root, also works on balancing the hormones. These sound like incredibly dramatic, wild names but many women do swear to the effectiveness of this form of therapy – probably the oldest form of medical treatment around.

She emphasises the importance of treating the adrenal glands to 'smooth out' the hormonal system. 'When ovaries have stopped producing oestrogen we can get the adrenals to produce their own similar hormones. The menopause can be a smooth experience if we can get the body to produce its own hormones.' Women who have never had a hot flush might find their bodies are doing that automatically.

'There must be a way for women with symptoms to get to the stage of those who never had any symptoms. If you take drugs you can never get your body back into balance,' she believes. We *don't* believe this!

Treatment can last for a few months to a couple of years. Anne thinks it is always preferable to see a herbalist rather than try to use these herbs yourself and we do agree with her here. 'Herbs can be very powerful substances and if you use them in the wrong way you might think they don't work or you might get an adverse effect, she says.'

Jill

Jill is a great believer in herbalism and feels it helped her a great deal through her menopause.

She had an early hysterectomy – at thirty-four – after 'no end of problems with a ruptured fallopian tube, ovarian cysts and endometriosis'. She had wanted children but was told it was a question of not surviving or losing her womb.

> The surgeon left me with a tiny bit of ovary which was healthy. He thought that would help me when I went through the menopause. At forty I was feeling the symptoms. I had hot flushes and mood swings, you name it I had it. My night sweats were terrible. I'd wake up wringing wet, I had to change my nightie, the sheets, everything. I'm normally calm and placid but I got depressed, fractious and I was tired all the time.

Jill says she suffered for an incredible twelve years.

> I thought it was never going to finish. The
> doctors kept saying they didn't want to put me
> on HRT as they didn't recognise it as safe then.
> They said there was nothing they could do. All
> the doctors I saw seemed to have the same
> attitude.

Her luck changed when she saw a BBC television
programme about herbalism. She decided it was worth a
try and contacted Anne.

> I felt I had nothing to lose. When my practitioner
> said, 'I can certainly help you,' I was overjoyed.
> She looked at my tongue and my eyes and
> checked my blood pressure and checked my
> knees and legs which had flared up and were
> swollen with arthritis. Then she gave me some
> herbs.
>   I think I felt worse before I felt better – but
> feeling worse was very short-term. That still
> happens now. It feels like the poison's coming out
> of my system. My body needed a total adjust-
> ment and that's what happened.

She also praises her herbalist's counselling skills and
says she believes that has helped her too.

> She's the sort of person who can draw you out of
> your shell. She puts you at ease straight away.
> There's no question of being herded in and out. I
> get time to talk about things and give her a
> complete picture.
>   I can't tell you how thankful I was to find
> someone at long last who could do something.

HOMOEOPATHY

The theory behind this is that a substance poisonous in large quantities can cure if taken in very small ones. The 'cures' will be given to you in the form of pills, capsules, sachets of powder or granules, or liquids.

Homoeopathic practitioners will want to know in great detail about your symptoms – even ones which don't seem to be remotely connected to the menopause. They will then put together a remedy which fits your requirements most closely. You may be asked about your personality and your character because these too will give the homoeopath clues as to your health and what you need.

The remedies are said to act as a signal which stimulates the body to self-heal. It involves the emotional, mental and physical aspects of the body.

As with herbalism, it's advisable to see a qualified practitioner who will be an expert and give you an appropriate remedy rather than trying to diagnose and treat yourself, but health shops and some chemists do have prepared remedies you can try. Remember not to take coffee or peppermint (even in toothpaste) while you're taking your remedy.

AROMATHERAPY

This relies upon natural aromatic essences concentrated from plants which are massaged into the skin or dropped into the bath. For menopausal problems, Daniele Ryman in *The Aromatherapy Handbook* suggests a combination of thyme (three drops), rosemary (two drops), basil (three drops), cypress (three drops) in an egg cup of soya oil to massage on to the tummy and the back of the neck. Do this yourself or get your partner or a friend to help. Or, instead, you could add to your bath either three drops of basil and three of cypress, three of thyme and three of rosemary or three of rosemary and three of basil.

HELPFUL ORGANISATIONS

United Kingdom

Amarant Trust, Grant House, 56–60 St John Street, London EC1M 4DT. Tel: 071 490 1644.

The menopause and HRT charity will provide lists of Well Woman and Menopause Clinics in your area if you send an SAE.

Also runs twenty-four-hour recorded telephone helplines, aiming to provide relevant, impartial and up-to-date information on HRT before you consult your doctor. The tapes are written by an expert gynaecologist Malcolm Whitehead. Calls cost, at cheap rate times, 5p for thirty-eight seconds.

Introduction and description of other lines 0836 400190
HRT, what is it and is it safe? 0836 400191
When should I start and how long should I stay on it? 0836 400192
Is it safe for everyone? 0836 400193
What are the possible side-effects? 0836 400194
How do I take it? 0836 400195
Where can I get it? 0836 400196
What checks and tests do I need before and while taking it? 0836 400197
What can it do for me and what are the short-term benefits? 0836 400198
Osteoporosis and other long-term benefits 0836 400199

Breast Care and Mastectomy Association, (i) 15–19 Britten Street, London SW3 3TZ. Tel: 071 867 8275; Help and information line: 071 867 1103. (ii) Suite 2–8, 65 Bath Street, Glasgow G2 2BX. Tel: 041 353 1050. (iii) 511 Lanark Road, Edinburgh EH14 5DQ. Tel: 031 458 5598.

Gives emotional support and practical information to women who have or fear they may have breast cancer.

British Acupuncture Association, 34 Alderney Street, London SW1 4EU. Tel: 071 834 1012 or 834 6229.
Will send a register of their members for £1.50.

British Association for Counselling, 1 Regent Place, Rugby CV21 2PJ. Tel: 0788 578328.
Provides details of counsellors near you, their specialised areas of work and their fees (if any).

British Complementary Medicine Association, St Charles Hospital, Exmoor Street, London W10 6DZ. Tel: 081 964 1205.

British Heart Foundation, 14 Fitzhardinge Street, London W1H 4DH. Tel: 071 935 0185.

British Homoeopathic Association, 27a Devonshire Street, London W1N 1RJ. Tel: 071 935 2163.

British Migraine Association, 178a High Road, Byfleet, Weybridge, Surrey. Tel: 0932 52468.

British Wheel of Yoga, 1 Hamilton Place, Boston Road, Sleaford, Lincs NG34 7ES. Tel: 0529 306851.

Council for Complementary and Alternative Medicine, 179 Gloucester Place, London NW1 6DX. Tel: 071 724 9103.

Council for Involuntary Tranquilliser Addiction (CITA), Cavendish House, Brighton Road, Waterloo, Liverpool L22 5NG. Tel: 051 525 2777.
Helps those addicted to tranquillisers.

Cruse, 126 Sheen Road, Richmond, Surrey TW9 1UR. Tel: 081 940 4818.
For bereavement counselling and care.

General Council and Register of Consultant Herbalists, Grosvenor House, 40 Seaway, Middleton-on-Sea, West Sussex PO22 7SA. Tel: 0243 586012.

General Council and Register of Osteopaths, 56 London Street, Reading, Berks RG1 4SQ. Tel: 0734 576585.

Hysterectomy Support Network, 3 Lynne Close, Green Street Green, Orpington, Kent BR6 6BS.

Institute of Complementary Medicine, PO Box 194, London SE16 1QZ. Tel: 071 237 5165.

Lifestyle Management, 13 Merton Hall Road, London SW19 3PP. Tel: 081 543 2086.
Has produced Stress Sensors to measure your stress level, a Stress Release Audio Tape to help you learn to relax, and other useful items.

Margaret Pyke Centre, 15 Bateman Buildings, Soho Square, London W1V 5TW. Tel: 071 734 9351.
Medical Director Professor John Guillebaud.

Mid-Life Matters, 32 Gwynne Road, Parkstone, Poole, Dorset BH12 2AS.
A service which provides herbal, vitamin and mineral alternatives to HRT.

Migraine Trust, 45 Great Ormond Street, London WC1N 3HZ. Tel: 071 278 2676.

National Association for Pre-Menstrual Syndrome, 33 Pilgrims Way West, Otford, Sevenoaks, Kent. Tel: 0732 459378; Information Line 0227 763133.

National Institute of Medical Herbalists, 9 Palace Gate, Exeter, Devon EX1 1JA. Tel: 0392 426022.

National Osteoporosis Society, PO Box 10, Radstock, Bath BA3 3YB. Tel: 0761 432472. Helpline 0761 431594.
Provides up-to-date information on osteoporosis/menopause/HRT/exercise; Produces eight booklets: including, Hormone Replacement Therapy, Exercise and Physiotherapy, your Cal-

cium Guide Book, HRT and Hysterectomy, How to Cope with Osteoporosis; Gives free confidential live helpline service for enquiries asking about the menopause, osteoporosis and HRT, the line being manned by specialist nurses. Free information pack and publication list – send a 1st class SAE.

Natural Therapeutic and Osteopathic Society, 14 Marford Road, Wheathampstead, Herts AL4 8AS. Tel: 0582 833950.

Parentline, Westbury House, 57 Hart Road, Thundersley, Essex SS7 3PD. Tel: 0268 757077.
Telephone helpline for parents under stress.

Parents Anonymous (London), 6 Manor Gardens, London N7 6LA. Tel: 071 263 8918.
Lifeline for distressed parents.

Relate (Marriage Guidance), Herbert Gray College, Little Church Street, Rugby, Warwickshire, CV21 3AP. Tel: 0788 573241.
Counselling help (you don't need to be married).

Relaxation for Living, 29 Burwood Park Road, Walton-on-Thames, Surrey KT12 5LH.
Runs relaxation classes, correspondence courses on relaxation and has leaflets, books and tapes.

The Society of Homoeopaths, 2 Artizan Road, Northampton NN1 4HU. Tel: 0604 21400.

Spectrum, 7 Endymion Road, London N4 1EE. Tel: 081 341 2277/340 0426.

Westminster Pastoral Foundation, 23 Kensington Square, London W8 5HN. Tel: 071 937 6956.
Provides counselling.

Women's Health Concern, 83 Earls Court Road, London W8 6LP. Tel: 071 938 3932.
Send an SAE for a free leaflet on HRT.

Women's Nationwide Cancer Control Campaign, Suna House, 128–130 Curtain Road, London EC2 3AR. Tel: 071 729 2229.
Offers information and advice on the screening and early detection of breast cancer.

Women's Therapy Centre, 6 Manor Gardens, London N7 6LA. Tel: 071 263 6200.
Please send an SAE when writing to any of the above organisations.

Canada

Acupuncture Foundation of Canada, 5 Roughfield Cr, Toronto ON M1S 4K3. Tel: (416) 291 4317.

Canadian Centre for Stress and Well-being, 181 University Avenue, 1202 Toronto ON M5H 3M7. Tel: (416) 363 6204.

Canadian Guidance and Counselling Association, 55 Parkdale Avenue, Ottawa ON K1Y 4G1. Tel: (613) 728 3281.

Canadian Institute of Stress, 1235 Bay Street, Toronto ON M5R 3K4. Tel: (416) 961 8575.

Canadian Osteopathic Aid Society, 575 Waterloo St, London ON N6B 2R2. Tel: (519) 439 5521.

Canadian Society of Homoeopathy, 87 Meadowland Drive W, Nepean ON K2G 2R9. Tel: (613) 723 1533.

Osteoporosis Society of BC, 203–2182 West 12th Avenue, Vancouver V6K 2N4. Tel: (604) 713 4997.

Osteoporosis Society of Canada, Suite 502, 76 St Claire Avenue West, Toronto, Ontario N4V 1N2. Tel: (416) 922 1358.

Ostop Ottawa, 220–1320 Richmond Road, Ottawa, Ontario K2B 8L3. Tel: (613) 596 9374.

Parental Stress Services – Parents Anonymous, PO Box 843, Burlington ON L7R 3Y7. Tel: (416) 333 3971.

Women's Counselling and Referral and Education Centre, 525 Bloor St W, Toronto ON M0M 0M0. Tel: (416) 534 7501.

Australia

Australian Acupuncture Association, 275 Moggill Road, Indooroopily, Queensland 4068. Tel: (07) 378 9377.

Australian Institute of Homoeopathy, 21 Bulah Close, Berowra Heights, New South Wales 2082. Tel: (02) 456 3602.

Australian Osteopathic Association, 4 Collins Street, Melbourne, Victoria. Tel: (03) 650 3736.

Canberra Marriage Guidance Council, 15 Hall Street, Lyneham, Canberra 2602. Tel: (06) 257 3273

Lifeline, 148 Lonsdale Street, Melbourne, Victoria 3000. Tel: (03) 662 1000.
Crisis telephone counselling, information and referral service.

Marriage Guidance Council of New South Wales, 5 Sera Street, Lane Cove, New South Wales 2066. Tel: (02) 418 8800.

Marriage Guidance Council of South Australia, 55 Hutt Street, Adelaide, South Australia 5000. Tel: (08) 223 4566.

Marriage Guidance Council of Western Australia, PO Box 1289, West Perth, Western Australia 6872. Tel: (09) 321 5801.

National Herbalists Association of Australia, PO Box 65, Kingsgrove, New South Wales 2208. Tel: (02) 502 2938.

Northern Territory Marriage Guidance Council, PO Box 4193, Darwin, Northern Territory 0801. Tel: (089) 816676.

Osteoporosis Foundation of Australia Incorporated, 100 Miller Street, 27th Floor, North Sydney, 2060 Australia. Tel: (02) 957 5162.

Queensland Marriage Guidance Council, 159 St Pauls Terrace, Brisbane, Queensland 4000. Tel: (07) 831 2005.

Tasmania Marriage Guidance Council, 306 Murray Street, Hobart, Tasmania 7000. Tel: (002) 313141.

Victoria Marriage Guidance Council, 46 Princess Street, Kew, Victoria 3101. Tel: (03) 853 5354.

Ireland

Irish Council for Complementary and Alternative Medicine, 87 North Circular Road, Dublin 7. Tel: (01) 388 196.

Marriage Counselling, 24 Grafton Street, Dublin. Tel: (01) 720 341.

Parents Under Stress, Carmichael House, North Brunswick Street, Dublin 7. Tel: (01) 733 500.

The Irish Family Planning Office, Books, Information and Education, 36–37 Lower Ormond Quay, Dublin 1. Tel: (01) 725 366.

Irish Family Planning Association, Unit 317, Level B, The Square Town Centre, Tallaght, Dublin 24. Tel: (01) 597 686.

Dublin Well-Woman Centre, 73 Lower Leeson Street, Dublin 2. Tel: (01) 610 083.

Well Woman Clinic, 35 Lower Liffey Street, Dublin 1. Tel: (01) 728 051.

National Association of Widows in Ireland, 12 Upper Ormond Quay, Dublin 7. Tel: (01) 770 977.
Helps widows adapt to their altered role in society. Offers counselling to newly bereaved widows, offers legal advice and organises social events and holidays.

AIM Group for Family Law Reform, AIM Centre, 64 Lower Mount Street, Dublin 2. Tel: (01) 616 478.

Branches at Social Services Centre, Dundalk, Co Louth. Tel: (042) 32848 (Friday mornings 10.30 – noon).

Waterford Resource Centre, Barrack Street, Waterford. Tel: (051) 74968.
Gives non directive counselling, legal information and a referral service to people with marriage and family problems.

New Zealand

Ministry of Women's Affairs, PO Box 10-049, Wellington. Tel: (04) 473 4112.

Health Department, PO Box 5013, Wellington. Tel: (04) 496 2000.

Marriage Guidance New Zealand, National Office, 150 Featherston Street, Wellington. Tel: (472) 8789 or 472 8107.
Call for your local branch.
These include: Wellington and Porirua, 8 Roxburgh Street, Mount Victoria. Tel: (385) 1729.

Hutt Valley, 14 Laings Road. Tel: (566) 4466.

Kapiti, PO Box 1602, Paraparaumu Beach. Tel: (298) 5655.

Auckland Central, Hampton Court, corner Wellesley and Federal Streets. Tel: (379) 0025.

Marriage and Couple Counselling Centre, 33 Owens Road, Epsom. Tel: (638) 7632.

Family Planning Association, National Office, 2nd Floor, Castrol House, corner of Dixon and Victoria Streets, Wellington. Tel: (384) 4349.

Cancerline, Cancer Society of New Zealand, PO Box 7125, Wellington South. Tel: (389) 5086.
Confidential information and advice service.

Acupuncture and Osteopathy and Holistic Centre, 21 Taharoto Road, Takapuna, Auckland. Tel: (489) 8219.

The Psychotherapy Centre, 7B Union Street, Dunedin. Tel: (479) 0996.

DRUGS USED IN HRT

COMBINED PREPARATIONS

Name	Formulations	Dosage
PREMPAKC (WYETH)	Natural conjugated equine oestrogens 0.625 mg (28 tabs) and 0.15 mg NG (12 tabs) [also 1.25 mg conjugated equine oestrogen (28 tabs) + 0.15 mg NG (12 tabs)].	1 oestrogen tablet for 16 days and 1 oestrogen + NG tablet for 12 days.
ESTRAPAK (CIBA)	Transdermal therapeutic patches 50 mcg Oestradiol per day (24 hrs) 8 patches. 1 mg tablets of NEA (12 tabs).	Apply new patch every 3–4 days. Tabs from day 15 to day 26.
NUVELLE (SCHERING)	E2V 2 mg (16 tabs) and E2V 2 mg + LNG 75 mcg (12 tabs)	1E2V tablet daily for the first 16 days then 1 combined table: daily for 12 days.
ESTRACOMBI (CIBA)	Transdermal therapeutic patches E2 50 mcg per 24 hrs (4 patches). E2 50 mcg plus NEA 250 mcg per 24 hrs (4 patches).	E2 patch twice weekly for 2 weeks, then combined patch twice weekly for 2 weeks.
CLIMAGEST (SANDOZ)	E2V 1 mg (16 tabs) and E2V 1 mg plus NEA 1 mg (12 tabs)	1 tablet daily in 28 day calendar pack.
LIVIAL ORGANON	Tibolone 2.5 mg tabs (28). Single molecule with oestrogen and progestogen activities.	1 tablet daily.
CYCLO-PROGYNOVA 1 mg (SCHERING)	E2V 1 mg (11 tabs) and E2V 1 mg plus LNG 0.25 mg (10 tabs.)	1 E2V tablet daily for 11 days, then 1 combined tab daily for 10 days followed by 7 tablet-free days.
CYCLO-PROGYNOVA 2 mg (SCHERING)	E2V 2 mg (11 tabs) and E2V 2 mg plus LNG 0.5 mg (10 tabs).	1 E2V tablet daily for 11 days then 1 combined tablet daily for 10 days followed by 7 tablet-free days.
TRISEQUENS FORTE NOVO-NORDISK	E2 4 mg + E3 2 mg (12 yellow tabs); E2 4 mg + E3 2 mg + NEA 1 mg (10 white tabs); E2 1 mg + E3 0.5 mg (8 red tabs).	1 tablet daily starting with yellow tabs.

OESTROGEN PREPARATIONS

Name	Formulations	Dosage
TRISEQUENS NOVO NORDISK	E2 2 mg + E3 1 mg (12 blue tabs); E2 2 mg + E3 1 mg + NEA 1 mg (10 white tabs); E2 1 mg + E3 0.5 mg (8 red tabs).	1 tablet daily starting with blue tablets.
PREMARIN (WYETH)	Conjugated equine oestrogens 0.625 mg or 1.25 mg or 2.5 mg tablets.	0.625–1.25 mg daily.
ESTRADERM (CIBA)	Transdermal therapeutic patches (8) releasing E2 25, 50, or 100 mcg per 24 hrs.	Apply new patch every 3 to 4 days.
PROGYNOVA (SCHERING)	E2V 1 mg or 2 mg tablets (21).	1 or 2 mg daily for 21 days then at least 7 tablet-free days.
HARMOGEN (ABBOTT)	Piperazine oestrone sulphate; 1.5 mg tablets.	1–3 tabs daily for 3 to 4 weeks, then 5 to 7 tablet-free days.
HORMONIN (SHIRE)	E3 0.27 mg + E1 1.4 mg + E2 0.6 mg tabs	1–2 tablets daily.
CLIMAVAL (SANDOZ)	E2V 1 mg or 2 mg tablets (28).	1–2 mg daily.
ZUMENON (DUPHAR)	Micronised E2 2 mg tablets (28).	1 tablet daily increasing if necessary to 2 daily.
OESTRADIOL IMPLANTS (ORGANON)	Fused implants of E2, 25, 50 or 100 mg	25–100 mg Reimplantation when symptoms recur, usually every 4–8 months.
ORTHO-DIENOESTROL (CILAG)	Dienoestrol .01% cream; 78 gms.	1 or 2 applicator doses (5 mg) intravaginally daily for 1 or 2 weeks. Maintenance; 1 applicator dose twice weekly.
ORTHO-GYNEST (CILAG)	Oestriol 0.5 mg pessary Oestriol .01%; Cream.	1 pessary inserted into the vagina every evening; or 1 applicator dose (5 mg) every evening. 1 pessary twice weekly or 1 applicator dose twice weekly for maintenance dose.

Name	Formulations	Dosage
PREMARIN CREAM (WYETH)	Conjugated oestrogens 0.625 mg per gm of non liquefying cream.	1–2 mgs topically or intravaginally daily for three weeks, then 1 week rest.
VAGIFEM (NOVO-NORDISK)	Oestrodiol; 25 mcg pessary.	1 pessary intravaginally daily for 2 weeks, then 1 pessary twice per week for three months.
OVESTIN (ORGANON)	Oestriol 0.1%; Cream.	1 applicator dose (0.5 mg) intravaginally for 3 weeks. Maintenance – 1 applicator dose twice weekly.

KEY

- NG = NORGESTREL
- LNG = LEVONORGESTREL   } i.e.:
- NEA = NORETHISTERONE ACETATE } Progestogens
- E1 = OESTRONE
- E2 = OESTRADIOL   } i.e.:
- E3 = OESTRIOL   } Oestrogens
- E2V = OESTRADIOL VALERATE

NHS Prescription Charges on HRT medicines:
There is often confusion over combined preparations when you may be asked to pay a double prescription charge. This is because there is a separate prescription charge for each medicine prescribed. Please ask your pharmacist if you have any queries.

INDEX